Malnutrition in Afghanistan

# Malnutrition in Afghanistan

*Scale, Scope, Causes, and Potential Response*

Emily Levitt, Kees Kostermans, Luc Laviolette,
and Nkosinathi Mbuya

**THE WORLD BANK**
**Washington, D.C.**

ISBN: 978-0-8213-8441-1
eISBN: 978-0-8213-8442-8
DOI: 10.1596/978-0-8213-8441-1

Cover photo: Emily Levitt

**Library of Congress Cataloging-in-Publication data has been applied for.**

# Contents

## Boxes

# Foreword

South Asia has by far the largest number of malnourished women and children, and no other region of the world has higher rates of malnutrition. Malnutrition in childhood is the biggest contributor to child mortality: a third of child deaths have malnutrition as an underlying cause. For the surviving children, malnutrition has lifelong implications because it severely reduces a child's ability to learn and to grow to his or her full potential. Malnutrition thus leads to less productive adults and weaker national economic performance. Therefore, the impact of malnutrition on a society's productivity and well being and a nation's long-term development is hard to underestimate.

For the South Asia Region of the World Bank, malnutrition is a key development priority, and in the coming years, the Bank intends to enhance dramatically its response to this challenge. As a first step, a series of country assessments such as this one are being carried out. These assessments will be used to reinforce the dialogue with governments and other development partners to scale up an evidence-based response against malnutrition. To succeed, we will need to address the problem comprehensively, which will require engaging several sectors.

This assessment of malnutrition in Afghanistan lays out the scale, scope, and causes of the problem. The scope is large—for example, 60 percent of children under five years of age are stunted. The assessment also indicates key elements of a potential response.

It will not be easy to respond in an effective way. However, as the Afghan proverb says, "There is a path to the top of even the highest mountain." We must reach this top together. The people of Afghanistan deserve nothing less.

Nick Krafft                              Julie McLaughlin
Country Director                         Sector Manager, Health
  for Afghanistan                          and Nutrition
The World Bank                           The World Bank

# Preface

Since late 2001, development partners—in particular, the United Nations Children's Fund (UNICEF) and the Food and Agriculture Organization of the United Nations (FAO)—have worked to create a strong infrastructure for nutrition in Afghanistan. From 2002 to 2005, an intensive investment was made in a Public Nutrition Department (PND) in the Ministry of Public Health, with in-office capacity-building support provided by UNICEF and Tufts University. Although based in the health sector, the PND coordinated actions across many sectors for nutrition through a network of task forces. This initiative led to a strong initial policy framework, skilled national staff, a network of Provincial Nutrition Officers, and a series of programs largely mainstreamed through sectoral programs. Since 2005, however, there have been challenges to sustaining the PND structure, including frequent staff changes in supporting institutions, competing international and national agendas, and loss of institutional memory. This book has the potential to contribute to a reversing of this trend, whereby activities in not only the health sector but also in other sectors relevant to nutrition will gain increased support and prominence in national development planning.

This comprehensive review also comes at a time when the Basic Package of Health Services (BPHS), a key platform for delivery of nutrition services, is in transition from a phase of expansion to a phase of quality improvement. The BPHS document includes many proposed nutrition interventions, but it is now time to act on them. The time is also ripe to take stock of the various models that have been developed and tested in different sectors in order to develop a cohesive multisectoral action plan for scaling up efforts to improve nutrition in Afghanistan. The intention of this book is to provide the background analysis for the development of an action plan.

This action plan would come at a time when development partner interest in nutrition is high. Subsequent to the 2008 publication in *The Lancet* of a series on maternal and child undernutrition, interest in nutrition among development partners and other development organizations has rapidly escalated. The analysis offered in this book is part of a broader effort within the World Bank's South Asia Region to scale up investments in nutrition, in recognition of the importance of good nutrition to well being, of economic growth and development, and of the large investment gaps in well-proven nutrition interventions.

# Acknowledgments

With funding from the Japanese Trust Fund and the World Bank's Central Contingency Fund, the South Asia Human Development Department undertook this assessment of the nutrition situation among Afghanistan's people. The task manager for this project was Kees Kostermans. Luc Laviolette and Nkosinathi Mbuya provided valuable inputs as part of the task team. Emily Levitt, consultant, was the main author of the report. Appreciated contributions to the planning of this Afghanistan multisectoral nutrition assessment and gap analysis were given by Harold Alderman, Yoichiro Ishihara, Dean Jolliffe, Alessandra Marini, Menno Mulder-Sibanda, John Newman, and Meera Shekar. Silvia Albert, Mohammed Khalid Khan, and Elfreda Vincent provided much-appreciated logistical assistance. Rose Esber edited the report and prepared it for publication. Thanks are also due to the many colleagues at the World Bank office in Kabul, Afghanistan, who supported this work and responded to queries with helpful information. Specifically, thanks are due to Ghulam Sayed, Tawab Hashemi, Hasib Karimzada, Asif Qurishi, and Hamidullah Abdullah.

This work would not have been possible without the dedicated efforts of the nutrition community in Afghanistan, which offered excellent support for this endeavor. These partners included those at the Public

Nutrition Department of the Ministry of Public Health; the Home Economics Department of the Ministry of Agriculture, Irrigation, and Livestock; the Ministry of Education; the Ministry of Rural Rehabilitation and Development; the Ministry of Labor, Social Affairs, Martyrs, and Disabled; the United Nations Children's Fund; the Food and Agriculture Organization of the United Nations; the World Food Programme; the World Health Organization; the Micronutrient Initiative; the United States Agency for International Development; the Basic Support for Institutionalizing Child Survival III Project; the Canadian International Development Agency; and numerous nongovernmental organizations. These institutions and their staffs provided time for extensive interviews, logistical support for arranging meetings with high-level government and other officials, and customarily excellent Afghan hospitality despite a challenging period in the country's history.

# Abbreviations

| | |
|---|---|
| ANDS | Afghanistan National Development Strategy |
| ANSA | Afghanistan National Standards Authority |
| ARDSS | Agriculture and Rural Development Sector Strategy |
| BASICS | Basic Support for Institutionalizing Child Survival (USAID Project) |
| BHC | basic health center |
| BMI | body mass index |
| BMS | breast milk substitute |
| BPHS | Basic Package of Health Services |
| CDC | Community Development Committee (of MRRD NSP) |
| CED | chronic energy deficiency |
| CGHN | Consultative Group on Health and Nutrition |
| CHC | comprehensive health center |
| CHW | community health worker |
| CMAM | community-based management of acute malnutrition |
| DPT3 | third dose of the diphtheria, pertussis, and tetanus vaccine |
| ESS | Education Sector Strategy |
| FAO | Food and Agriculture Organization of the United Nations |

| | |
|---|---|
| FHAG | family health action group |
| GAP | Global Action Plan (for Nutrition) |
| HED | Home Economics Department (of the Ministry of Agriculture, Irrigation, and Livestock) |
| HLP | Horticulture and Livestock Project |
| HMIS | Health Management Information System |
| HNSS | Health and Nutrition Sector Strategy |
| IFA | iron and folic acid |
| IMCI | Integrated Management of Childhood Illness |
| IYCF | infant and young child feeding |
| KAP | knowledge, attitudes, and practices |
| LBW | low birth weight |
| MAIL | Ministry of Agriculture, Irrigation, and Livestock |
| MDD | micronutrient deficiency disorder |
| MDG | Millennium Development Goals |
| MI | Micronutrient Initiative |
| MMR | maternal mortality rate |
| MOC | Ministry of Commerce |
| MOLSAMD | Ministry of Labor, Social Affairs, Martyrs, and Disabled |
| MOPH | Ministry of Public Health |
| MRRD | Ministry of Rural Rehabilitation and Development |
| NADF | National Agriculture Development Framework |
| NCHS | National Center for Health Statistics |
| NGO | nongovernmental organization |
| NIDs | National Immunization Days |
| NNS | National Nutrition Survey (2004) |
| NRVA | National Risk and Vulnerability Assessment |
| NSP | National Solidarity Program |
| PCC | Provincial Coordination Committee |
| PND | Public Nutrition Department (of the Ministry of Public Health) |
| PNO | Provincial Nutrition Officer |
| PNPS | Public Nutrition Policy and Strategy |
| PPA | performance-based partnership agreement |
| RuWatSIP | MRRD Rural Water, Sanitation, and Irrigation Program |
| SFP | Supplementary Feeding Program |
| SPSS | Social Protection Sector Strategy |
| STAR | Strategies for Trauma Awareness and Resilience (program) |
| SUN | Scaling Up Nutrition (initiative) |

| | |
|---|---|
| TFU | therapeutic feeding unit |
| TOT | training-of-trainers (approach) |
| U2 | under two years of age |
| U5 | under five years of age |
| UN | United Nations |
| UNICEF | United Nations Children's Fund |
| USAID | United States Agency for International Development |
| VAD | vitamin A deficiency |
| WFP | World Food Programme |
| WHO | World Health Organization |

# Overview

## Nutrition Situation in Afghanistan

Levels of child undernutrition in Afghanistan are very high. The 2004 National Nutrition Survey (NNS), using the World Health Organization (WHO) updated references, found that 60.5 percent of children under the age of five were stunted and 33.7 percent were underweight (MOPH and others 2009). The stunting levels are among the highest in the world. Acute undernutrition (wasting) in children under five was 8.7 percent, lower than would be expected for a country experiencing protracted conflict, but these wasting levels remain very high in the first few years of life (18.1 percent in children 1–2 years). Micronutrient and anemia data are largely available from subsamples of less remote areas, unless otherwise noted, and are therefore taken as underestimates. The prevalence of anemia is 38 percent in children under five and 50 percent in children 6 to 24 months old. Both iron and iodine deficiency affect 72 percent of children under five. No data for zinc are available, but estimates (between 60.5 and 72 percent) can be made from combining the stunting estimate and that of iron deficiency because zinc deficiency typically manifests with these conditions. Scurvy (clinical vitamin C deficiency) has been reported in up to 10 percent of households in some remote, mountainous provinces (Cheung and others 2003). No national data on vitamin A are

1

available for children, but 9.9 percent maternal night blindness suggests a significant deficiency problem in the population.

Maternal undernutrition is also a significant challenge. The 2004 NNS (MOPH and others 2009) found that 20.9 percent of nonpregnant women of reproductive age had chronic energy deficiency (body mass index less than18.5). Hence, chronic energy deficiency is considered a problem of high prevalence according to WHO standards. The prevalence of iodine deficiency in pregnant and nonpregnant women was at least 75 percent. Iron deficiency was 48.4 percent and anemia 25 percent among nonpregnant women. Women who were literate or had access to at least primary education were less likely to be undernourished and to have micronutrient deficiencies. A high incidence of birth defects (neural tube defects) in Kabul hospitals also may suggest folate deficiency in the population, particularly among women.

The critical window for nutrition intervention in children is from the day of conception to 24 months of age to avert irreversible damage to growth and development, as well as increased morbidity and mortality risk. Because maternal, infant, and child mortality rates in Afghanistan are among the highest in the world, improving the nutritional status of these groups is imperative. Intervention prior to pregnancy and until a child is 24 months of age is important to improve their overall health and future economic productivity.

Public investments in nutrition are critical to support economic and social development and to provide increased stability supportive of national security (Pinstrup-Andersen and Shimokawa 2008). Malnutrition reduces a country's gross domestic product by 2 to 3 percent (World Bank 2006). Interventions to address malnutrition have been selected as 5 of the top 10 best investments for national development by the Copenhagen Consensus 2008. The Millennium Development Goals (MDGs) also highlight reductions in malnutrition as the first goal, and nutrition is a factor in reaching several other goals as well.

## Conceptual Framework

This situation analysis of nutrition in Afghanistan was conducted using the following two frameworks:

- *Determinants of undernutrition.* The United Nations Children's Fund (UNICEF) conceptual framework for understanding the causes of malnutrition is applied to analyze the importance of (a) food security,

(b) health and health services, (c) health environment, and (d) care for women and children as key determinants of undernutrition. The degree of general nutrition awareness in the population is also examined.

- *Five pillars of the Global Action Plan:* The World Bank and other partners are considering a framework arising from the Global Action Plan for Nutrition, which has been renamed the Scaling Up Nutrition (SUN) initiative. This framework, which aims to prioritize and cost out nutrition interventions in developing countries, was also used to structure the analysis. The following five pillars, considered to be essential elements of comprehensive national action on nutrition, form the basis of the analysis:
  - *Pillar 1:* Nutrition is recognized as foundational to national development.
  - *Pillar 2:* Adequate local capacity is built and supported to design and execute effective nutrition policies and programs.
  - *Pillar 3:* Cost-effective, direct nutrition interventions are scaled up, where applicable.
  - *Pillar 4:* Determinants of undernutrition are addressed through multisectoral approaches.
  - *Pillar 5:* Coordinated support for nutrition is provided by development partners (including funding for advocacy, communications, and research).

## Determinants of Undernutrition in Afghanistan

All key determinants of undernutrition interact to create the current situation in Afghanistan:

- Afghanistan faces a serious food security challenge, with 28 percent of Afghan households having inadequate caloric intake and at least a third of households consuming diets with inadequate food diversity, according to national surveys.

- Insufficient health services remain a determinant of undernutrition because the prevalence of illness in the population remains very high. Although 65 percent of households now have access within two hours of walking to a Basic Package of Health Services (BPHS) facility, up from 9 percent in 2000, many households still do not have the means to make optimal use of these facilities (for example, because of cost, transportation, or cultural constraints).

- The health environment in Afghanistan remains a significant cause of undernutrition. Seventy-three percent of households still lack access to safe drinking water, and 95 percent lack access to improved sanitation. Hygiene practices are also a concern, because hand washing with soap is not yet a mainstream practice.

- Inadequate care for women and children is also a significant cause of undernutrition in the country. Women have limited influence over how resources are spent and what foods are purchased. The response to the special needs of women and children has also not been adequate: use of prenatal care and contraceptives remains low. Despite the very high levels of maternal underweight (20.9 percent of women have low BMI), no supplementation programs for women are available through the health system (food or multiple micronutrient interventions). Deworming is infrequent although available. Inadequate infant and young child feeding (IYCF) practices represent an important area for intervention. Exclusive breastfeeding is thought to be extremely rare, whereas predominant breastfeeding (which allows for some liquids and ritual practices) more accurately describes the Afghan custom. Only about one-third of children are given complementary foods at the proper time of six months.

## Political Economy, Institutional and Implementation Arrangements, and Capacity to Address Undernutrition

Pillars 1 and 2 of the Global Action Plan addressed institutional and implementation arrangements, as well as capacity considerations.

### Pillar 1: Is Nutrition Recognized as Foundational to National Development?

The Afghanistan National Development Strategy (ANDS), the country's poverty reduction strategy, is designed to achieve all of the Millennium Development Goals. Within the ANDS, two sector strategies are chiefly responsible for addressing undernutrition: the Health and Nutrition Sector Strategy and the Agriculture and Rural Development Sector Strategy. Despite these supportive policy statements, support for nutrition within the corresponding line ministries is still weak, as indicated by the low positioning of nutrition-related departments within the organizational structures and low funding priority given to nutrition programs. The critical sectors, therefore, do not view nutrition as foundational to national development. Research in 2006 and 2007 found that this low salience is less because of lack of interest than because of unfamiliarity with the prevalence of the problem in Afghanistan, lack of awareness of evidence-based relationships between undernutrition and morbidity and mortality, and bias of development partners (and corresponding funding agendas) to other issues.

The two government departments directly dedicated to nutrition are the Public Nutrition Department (PND) of the Ministry of Public Health (MOPH) and the Home Economics Department (HED) of the Ministry of Agriculture, Irrigation, and Livestock (MAIL). The MOPH now funds a core PND national staff and a cadre of 34 provincial nutrition officers (one per province). An evidence-based MOPH Public Nutrition Policy and Strategy has existed in Afghanistan since 2003, but there have been challenges related to its implementation. The revised Public Nutrition Strategy (2009–13) focuses largely on direct nutrition interventions through the health sector, making mention of the critical links to other related sectors supportive of nutrition. A need remains for an overarching, national nutrition coordination mechanism with authority over sectoral activities. The MAIL's HED plays a strong role in promoting improved child feeding practices and household food security. The HED is also hiring provincial-level home economics officers, who are to work in collaboration with the provincial nutrition officers to scale up nutrition activities.

The following ministries also have important nutrition-related functions:

- *Ministry of Rural Rehabilitation and Development.* This ministry is responsible for food security surveillance (for example, through the National Risk and Vulnerability Assessment), improved access to safe drinking water, and improved sanitation and hygiene.
- *Ministry of Labor, Social Affairs, Martyrs, and Disabled.* This ministry implements social protection programs for vulnerable families (often female-headed households with small children). Reducing child underweight is a goal highlighted in the ANDS Social Protection Sector Strategy.
- *Ministry of Education.* This ministry collaborates with the MAIL's HED and the Food and Agriculture Organization of the United Nations (FAO) on promoting nutrition through the schools. A separate Healthy Schools Initiative does not currently include a nutrition promotion component (apart from deworming activities), but the Ministry of Education has begun a dialogue with the MAIL's HED to scale up the

school-based nutrition programs and possibly link them to the Healthy Schools Initiative.

- *Ministry of Higher Education.* This ministry includes some nutrition topics in the medical curriculum and is exploring options with development partners to expand nutrition training.
- *Ministry of Women's Affairs.* This ministry collaborates in nutrition promotion through women's groups (for example, by providing nutrition education in the context of literacy courses).
- *Ministry of Commerce.* This ministry has links with the private sector, especially in relation to food fortification (domestic production as well as importation). It supports the Afghanistan National Standards Authority, which aims to monitor food safety and quality.
- *Ministry of Justice.* All legal issues related to nutrition are coordinated through this ministry (for example, issues related to the enforcement of the Code of Marketing of Breast Milk Substitutes, maternity leave, and workplace access to nurseries for overall child care as well as to assist breastfeeding mothers).
- *Ministry of Religious Affairs.* This ministry provides nutrition promotion messages to religious leaders for dissemination to the general public.

### Pillar 2: Is Adequate Local Capacity Built and Supported to Design and Execute Effective Nutrition Policies and Programs?

The two government departments described earlier (the MOPH's PND and the MAIL's HED) were examined with the capacity assessment framework developed by Potter and Brough (2004). This assessment uses a four-tier hierarchy of capacity-building needs:

1. Structures, systems, and roles
2. Staff and facilities
3. Skills
4. Tools

Tier 1 (structures, systems, and roles) forms the base of the capacity structure, with each successive tier building on the one before it. Overall, the review found that though important efforts have been made to build the capacity of the two main government departments, significant capacity gaps exist.

The PND has increasing personnel capacity relating to nutrition skills and knowledge of technical content. Policies and programs have been developed with outside technical support that are based on best practices and evidence. The capacity gaps facing the PND include components of the other eight types of capacities, because these capacities are largely outside the PND's control. The eight types are role, systems, structures, support service, workload, supervisory, facility, and performance capacities. In brief, the PND has received intensive capacity-building support from international partners, yet greater support is needed to sustain the structure that was set up. Additional management and financial management trainings have also been requested.

The HED is in a different situation. It is largely the beneficiary of a grant provided to FAO, which includes the HED as a direct beneficiary. FAO supports the HED in building capacity and providing technical support to policies and programs. The few gaps that have been identified currently relate to workload, supervisory, facility, and performance capacities. As personnel capacity increases, the HED will need to achieve greater sustainability without FAO's extensive, direct support, which may end after December 2010.

Although it will be important to continue to build capacity within the MOPH and MAIL, addressing capacity gaps in the Ministry of Rural Rehabilitation and Development—particularly to enable the acceleration of scale-up of safe drinking water and improved sanitation and hygiene—will also be critical. Addressing the capacity of the overall nutrition system (that is, the national capacity to plan for nutrition across multiple sectors, implement that plan in each sector, and then review results and lessons learned on a multisectoral basis) is similarly important. Elements of that system are currently in place (for example, for policy formulation), but some capacity gaps exist (program planning, execution, and results monitoring and review). The capacity of the government to harness the resources and capacity of the private sector in Afghanistan to improve nutrition (through, for example, marketing of nutrition products, promotion of nutrition-enhancing behaviors, and regulation of fortification of foods) will also need to be enhanced.

## Programs, Gaps, and Opportunities

Pillars 3 and 4 deal with programs, gaps, and opportunities.

### Pillar 3: Are Cost-Effective, Direct Nutrition Interventions Scaled Up?

Overall, though some success has been achieved in scaling up direct nutrition interventions in Afghanistan (for example, vitamin A supplementation), much more work remains to be done to scale up a well-proven basic set of direct nutrition interventions.

There are no major mismatches between policies for nutrition in Afghanistan and international best practice. However, very few interventions are operating at a significant scale nationally. The MOPH's BPHS provides many of the interventions recommended by the 2008 *Lancet* series on maternal and child undernutrition, but most of them need to be significantly scaled up. The available interventions include

- Prepregnancy and maternal nutrition:
  - Iron and folic acid supplementation through prenatal and postnatal (three months postpartum) care services. Prenatal care coverage is 36 percent.
  - Vitamin A supplements for postpartum women provided through immunization activities. Coverage is less than 25 percent.
  - Free deworming treatment at all levels of the health system. Use of such services is very low.
  - Provision of insecticide-treated bed nets in malaria-prone areas. Adequate support exists.
- Infant and young child nutrition:
  - High coverage of vitamin A supplementation (coverage for two doses annually is at more than 90 percent) through polio immunization campaigns, as well as through facilities. An alternative program model is needed because campaigns may eventually be phased out.
  - Largely facility-based promotion of optimal breastfeeding and complementary feeding practices. Such promotion is provided through, for example, Integrated Management of Child Illness (IMCI) mother care, prenatal care, and hospitals, as well as through community health workers (CHWs).
  - A pilot growth promotion program that provides a platform for promotion of maternal and child nutrition and health, including IYCF. The program is currently in five provinces.
  - Anemia treatment through an IMCI regimen in BPHS facilities. Data are unavailable on iron supplement use for children under two.
  - Diarrhea treatment with oral rehydration solution and zinc. In a revised policy, there is a need for support to scale up provision of zinc supplements.
  - Prevention and treatment of acute undernutrition through therapeutic feeding units and supplementary feeding programs in areas

with high prevalence. Therapeutic feeding units need greater support to manage their caseload.

The MAIL's HED plays a lead role in promoting improved complementary feeding practices at the community level. Training-of-trainers strategies
are used and scaled up through various community platforms, largely
involving women. Activities are supported in 5 provinces with FAO support, but the HED staff is trained and available in an additional 12 provinces
to scale up these efforts. This program's influence should be evaluated.

Food fortification programs in collaboration with the private sector
include the following:

- *Flour fortification.* The eight large wheat-flour millers in Afghanistan are
  participating in fortification efforts with support from the Micronutrient Initiative (MI) and the World Food Programme. However, the large
  mills reach mainly consumers in urban and peri-urban areas and currently provide fortified wheat flour to only about 8 percent of the
  urban population.

- *Universal salt iodization and double-fortified salt.* Since 2003, universal
  salt iodization has been a public-private sector partnership of the
  MOPH with support from UNICEF and, more recently, MI. Coverage
  is currently estimated at 50 percent. Imports of foreign salt have been
  banned because Afghanistan has the production capacity to supply
  the entire population with iodized salt. This decision to ban salt imports has put in jeopardy progress achieved on salt iodization because
  domestic salt is mined using crude approaches that lead to contamination with mud and possibly heavy metals such as lead. Consumers
  view the darker salt as "dirty" and prefer to purchase smuggled salt
  from neighboring countries. Double fortification of salt with iron as
  well as iodine will require additional support and is being explored by
  MI, UNICEF, and the MOPH, given successes in India.

- *Oil and ghee fortification.* MI, UNICEF, and the MOPH are exploring
  legislation to support importation of oil and ghee fortified with vitamin A. Current imports may label products as fortified, but studies
  have shown that such labeling is often false.

- *Multiple micronutrient powders.* Emergency programs currently include
  multiple micronutrient powders that are provided on a limited scale

to children, but there is no routine provision through the BPHS or private sector channels.

### Pillar 4: Are Determinants of Undernutrition Addressed through Multisectoral Approaches?

Although some progress has been made in harnessing the potential of various sectors to improve nutrition in Afghanistan, much more needs to be done:

- *Food security and related surveillance activities* are being supported by the MAIL, but current activities are not well coordinated. The MAIL's HED is involved in many food security interventions, which should be reinforced and scaled up.
- *Access to health services* has improved significantly, with 65 percent of the population now having some access to health services. However, various weather-related, geographic, economic, and cultural constraints limit greater access, particularly for women, and as a result health and nutrition indicators are less than optimal.
- *The health environment* still presents a significant challenge. Coverage rates for safe water and improved sanitation are very low, and current demand far exceeds available funding.
- *Care for women and children* also needs to be improved. The revised BPHS has included a stronger component for mental health support. Maternal depression is associated with poor infant feeding practices and "insufficient milk" syndrome. Despite the newly designed infrastructure for mental health, funding allocations to roll out these services are still limited.
- *Nutrition education* is still relatively weak. Nutrition promotion activities to the general public have focused on specific topics (such as iodized salt and breastfeeding). Basic nutrition concepts and guidelines are not well understood at both community and government levels and even within the medical community, which is the main source of nutrition advice to households.

### Pillar 5: Is Coordinated Support for Nutrition Provided by Development Partners?

Although nutrition is a topic of some of the coordination groups, nutrition issues are not given sufficient prominence; hence, coordination between development partners has been less than optimal. The Consultative Group on Health and Nutrition (CGHN), which supports the Health and Nutrition Sector Strategy, includes participation from development partners and meets regularly at the MOPH. Nutrition is periodically an agenda item, but it is not a major focus of the development partners. The revised BPHS includes increased support for nutrition, and specific programs are periodically discussed in the CGHN. A Nutrition Cluster meets regularly—largely with government, United Nations (UN) and nongovernment organization (NGO) participation—but focuses on nutrition in emergencies. Development partners meet as needed to address nutrition issues in a Nutrition Task Force, which is facilitated by the MOPH PND. Participants in the Nutrition Task Force are largely the same implementers as those of the Nutrition Cluster (that is, government ministries, the UN, and NGOs). Most coordination mechanisms currently exist through the UN system. An Agriculture Task Force has been formed as well, with some attention to nutrition and food security issues.

## Recommendations

Recommendations are provided in accordance with the pillar structure originating in the Global Action Plan for Nutrition.

### Pillar 1: Nutrition Is Recognized as Foundational to National Development

The following recommendations will help make nutrition foundational to national development:

- Creation of a National Cross-Cutting Nutrition Strategy modeled on other cross-cutting strategies in the ANDS system should be considered. Appropriate high-level contributors should be identified, and formation of a high-level multisectoral coordination committee (for example, a consultative group) dedicated to nutrition should be considered.
- Advocacy is required by the nutrition community and its development partners to increase valuation of nutrition as a national investment, particularly in the health and agriculture sectors.
- The Ministry of Labor, Social Affairs, Martyrs, and Disabled (MOLSAMD) shows strong support for nutrition and nutrition-related MDGs through its Social Protection Sector Strategy. The MOLSAMD should be included as a stronger partner in nutrition programming.

## Pillar 2: Adequate Local Capacity Is Built and Supported to Design and Execute Effective Nutrition Policies and Programs

The following recommendations will assist in local capacity building and support:

- Support is needed for some government staff members to receive either distance-learning training or training abroad at least at a master's degree level in modern nutrition science, policies, and programs (including research methods).
- Support is needed for a nutrition degree program at an Afghan university or health institute (for example, Kabul Medical University or Kabul University Faculty of Agriculture).
- The issue of inadequate control over nutrition funding by the government of Afghanistan must be addressed.
- Resources must be ensured to meet basic capacity needs such as transportation for coordinating and monitoring, communications for supervision, and meeting spaces that are suitable for women.

## Pillar 3: Cost-Effective, Direct Nutrition Interventions Are Scaled Up, Where Applicable

Recommendations for scale-up through the BPHS are as follows:

- Breastfeeding counselor training should be scaled up through the MOPH's PND national and provincial staffs.
- Access and use of women's health care (such as prenatal care, iron and folic acid supplementation, vitamin A supplementation, deworming, and birth spacing) need to be improved. Conditional programs (such as cash transfers and food supplements for underweight women) should be considered.
- Community-level programming can be improved through mechanisms such as CHW support groups (for example, family health action groups) for IYCF, diarrhea management (oral rehydration solution or zinc), deworming, referrals for immunization and treatment of infections, early identification of malnourished children and admission to community-based management of acute malnutrition, and maternal health care. Zinc should be provided in the remaining BPHS provinces.
- Development of a cadre of community nutrition workers similar to models adopted successfully in Nepal and Pakistan should be considered.

- Hygiene should be promoted through BPHS facilities and community support structures.

The following recommendations would be accomplished through agriculture and broader sectoral partnerships:

- Complementary feeding (and broad IYCF) promotion activities should be scaled up through multiple community-level platforms that reach women by using trained and available staff members of the MAIL's HED.
- Nutrition promotion activities should be combined with a package of activities to improve household food security in food insecure areas, because evidence shows greater likelihood of success when combined interventions are used in such areas.
- The HED's School-Based Nutrition Promotion program should be scaled up as a strategy to reach girls before marital engagement. A component on nutrition throughout the life course should be included for girls and, if possible, boys, because boys will be future providers and do most of the food purchasing.

These recommendations can be implemented through public-private partnerships:

- Zinc supplementation coverage should be expanded through the private sector medical community, because many Afghans do not use government health services. Quality control of other nutrition activities (iron and folic acid supplementation) should be scaled up through private sector medical services.
- A market feasibility study of multiple micronutrient powders should be conducted to address anemia and other deficiencies through commercial channels.
- The bottleneck of the contaminated domestic salt supply *urgently* needs to be addressed through provision of a salt purification facility and other programmatic inputs to improve the quality and sustainability of salt iodization.
- The double fortification of salt with both iron and iodine to address anemia needs to be pursued, particularly in rural areas that will not be reached by wheat flour milled by large mills.
- Support should be provided for the formation of a flour millers' association in Afghanistan for coordination, quality control, and mutual

accountability. Support should continue to be provided to wheat-flour millers to fortify flour milled in Afghanistan. The possibility of fortifying flour that is milled in neighboring countries (especially Pakistan) and imported into Afghanistan ought to be explored.

- Legislation is needed for fortified products and quality control and enforcement measures.

### Pillar 4: Determinants of Undernutrition Are Addressed through Multisectoral Approaches

Recommendations that can be implemented through the MAIL are as follows:

- Support is required to strengthen and coordinate food security surveillance activities.
- The HED's training-of-trainers activities through various community platforms should be evaluated to determine how they can best be scaled up.
- Food security–related outcome indicators should be included in horticulture and livestock program evaluations. Requiring nutrition indicators as a condition of funding ought to be considered.

The following recommendations can be implemented through the Ministry of Rural Rehabilitation and Development:

- The ministry's Rural Water, Sanitation, and Irrigation Program needs support to meet the high demand for promotion activities related to safe drinking water and improved sanitation and hygiene.
- Support for the National Solidarity Program must be continued because the top request from communities is still for safe drinking water. Nutrition-tagged funding could be provided through Rural Water, Sanitation, and Irrigation Program for the National Solidarity Program's water, sanitation, and hygiene requests.

These recommendations can be carried out through the MOLSAMD:

- Social protection programs to vulnerable households should be supported. These programs should include nutrition promotion as a component of a broader food security intervention (such as training provided by the MAIL's HED with respect to cash transfer, food for work, food for education, and food security and income generation).

- Links under Pillar 3 should be considered with the MOLSAMD's kindergartens and orphanages.

## Pillar 5: Coordinated Support for Nutrition Is Provided by Development Partners

An improved mechanism is required to adequately coordinate the varied multisectoral activities related to nutrition.

## References

Cheung, Edith, Roya Mutahar, Fitsum Assefa, Mija-Tesse Ververs, Shah Mahmood Nasiri, Annalies Borrel, and Peter Salama. 2003. "An Epidemic of Scurvy in Afghanistan: Assessment and Response." *Food and Nutrition Bulletin* 24 (3): 247–55.

MOPH (Ministry of Public Health), UNICEF (United Nations Children's Fund), CDC (Centers for Disease Control and Prevention), National Institute for Research on Food and Nutrition–Italy, and Tufts University. 2009. *2004 Afghanistan National Nutrition Survey.* Atlanta: CDC.

Pinstrup-Andersen, Per, and Satoru Shimokawa. 2008. "Do Poverty and Poor Health and Nutrition Increase the Risk of Armed Conflict Onset?" *Food Policy* 33 (6): 513–20.

Potter, Christopher, and Richard Brough. 2004. "Systemic Capacity Building: A Hierarchy of Needs." *Health Policy and Planning* 19 (5): 336–54.

World Bank. 2006. *Repositioning Nutrition as Central to Development: A Strategy for Large-Scale Action.* Washington, DC: World Bank.

# CHAPTER 1

# Introduction

## Rationale

The purpose of this assessment is to provide the basis for future World Bank operational support to fight malnutrition in Afghanistan. It aims to (a) review the size, severity, and key determinants of undernutrition; (b) review the present capacity, institutional, and implementation arrangements in the public and private sectors to address undernutrition; (c) identify gaps and suggest options for support by the government of Afghanistan and development partners to enhance the country's response to undernutrition; and (d) outline the needs for new institutional arrangements, organizational (system) development, and technical and management capacity to address identified gaps in the response.

Malnutrition—specifically undernutrition—is endemic in Afghanistan. Public investments in nutrition are critical to support economic and social development and provide increased stability supportive of national security (Pinstrup-Andersen and Shimokawa 2008). Malnutrition reduces a country's gross domestic product by 2 to 3 percent (World Bank 2006). Interventions to address malnutrition have been selected as 5 of the top 10 best investments for national development by the Copenhagen Consensus 2008 (table 1.1).[1] The Millennium Development Goals also

**Table 1.1    Nutrition and the Copenhagen Consensus 2008**

| Solution (in order of most cost-effective to least) | Challenge |
|---|---|
| 1. Micronutrient supplements for children (vitamin A and zinc) | **Malnutrition** |
| 2. The Doha development agenda | Trade |
| 3. Micronutrient fortification (iron and salt iodization) | **Malnutrition** |
| 4. Expanded immunization coverage for children | Diseases |
| 5. Biofortification | **Malnutrition** |
| 6. Deworming and other nutrition programs at school | **Malnutrition** and education |
| 7. Lowering of the price of schooling | Education |
| 8. Increase in and improvement of girls' schooling | Women |
| 9. Community-based nutrition promotion | **Malnutrition** |
| 10. Provision of support for women's reproductive role | Women |

*Source:* Results of the 2008 Copenhagen Consensus, http://www.copenhagenconsensus.com/Home.aspx.

highlight reductions in malnutrition as the first goal, and nutrition is a factor in the achievement of several other goals (table 1.2).

### Significant Improvements in Child Health Indicators

For the past three decades, Afghanistan has experienced a prolonged civil war that has destroyed the country's infrastructure; fragmented institutions; and left most parts of the country without health, education, and sanitation facilities. However, during the past seven years, the country has achieved considerable results in a challenging context. Progress in the health sector has been particularly remarkable, most of which can be attributed to strong Ministry of Public Health (MOPH) leadership, sound public health policies, innovative service delivery models, and a strong focus on monitoring of performance. The effect of this progress on child health outcomes has been encouraging.

The National Risk and Vulnerability Assessment (NRVA) 2007/08 found that the infant mortality rate has declined from 2001 estimates of 165 per 1,000 live births to 111 per 1,000 live births. Under-five (U5) mortality has also declined from 257 per 1,000 live births to 161 per 1,000 live births (CSO 2009). The NRVA 2007/08 showed that the percentage of children receiving the third dose of the diphtheria, pertussis, and tetanus vaccine (DPT3) coverage had increased to 43 percent, and full immunization increased to 37 percent (CSO 2009). Nevertheless, the U5 mortality rate in Afghanistan is still higher than the average for low-income countries. Moreover, the low vaccination coverage (for example, DPT3) still

**Table 1.2    Nutrition and the Millennium Development Goals**

| Goal | Nutrition effect |
|---|---|
| Goal 1: Eradicate extreme poverty and hunger. | • Malnutrition represents the nonincome face of poverty.<br>• Malnutrition erodes human capital through irreversible and intergenerational effects on cognitive and physical development.<br>• Iron intake can reduce anemia, leading to greater productivity and earning potential.<br>• Intake of iodized salt reduces iodine deficiency disorders, thereby increasing learning ability and intellectual potential, leading ultimately to better-educated citizens earning higher wages.<br>• Zinc reduces stunting and severity of diarrhea among children. |
| Goal 2: Achieve universal primary education. | • Malnutrition affects the chances that a child will go to school, stay in school, and perform well.<br>• Intake of iodized salt prevents the loss of 10 to 15 IQ points, thereby improving cognitive development and learning potential in salt-deficient populations.<br>• Iron intake by young children improves cognitive development and learning potential.<br>• Zinc intake reduces the frequency and severity of diarrhea, thus decreasing the number of school days lost.<br>• Vitamin A intake prevents child blindness.<br>• Folic acid consumption prevents disability caused by neural tube defects. |
| Goal 3: Promote gender equality and empower women. | • Antifemale biases in access to food, health, and care resources may result in malnutrition.<br>• Addressing malnutrition empowers women. |
| Goal 4: Reduce child mortality. | • Malnutrition is directly or indirectly associated with most child deaths, and it is the major contributor to the burden of disease in the developing world.<br>• Vitamin A supplementation twice per year has the potential to reduce child mortality among deficient populations by as much as 23%.<br>• Zinc intake can reduce child mortality by 4%<br>• Consumption of iodized salt lowers rates of miscarriage, stillbirth, and neonatal death. |
| Goal 5: Improve maternal health. | • Maternal health is compromised by malnutrition, which is associated with most major risk factors for maternal mortality. Maternal stunting and iron deficiency particularly pose serious problems. |
| Goal 6: Combat HIV/AIDS, malaria, and other diseases. | • Malnutrition may increase the risk of HIV transmission, compromise the effectiveness of antiretroviral therapy, and hasten the onset of full-blown AIDS and premature death.<br>• Malnutrition increases the chances of tuberculosis infection resulting in disease, and it also reduces malarial survival rates. |

*Sources:* Updated from World Bank 2006 and MOPH 2009.

reflects the population's poor physical access to health facilities, with more than 60 percent of Afghans living more than one hour's walk away from a health facility.

### Very High Child Undernutrition Rates and Chronic Undernutrition Levels

Notwithstanding improvements in health indicators, the indicators of child and maternal undernutrition still remain grim. Using the new World Health Organization (WHO) references, the 2004 National Nutrition Survey (NNS) found 60.5 percent of U5 children to be stunted (that is, to be suffering from chronic undernutrition) and 33.7 percent to be underweight (MOPH and others 2009). The wasting prevalence for U5 children was 8.7 percent—below expectations for a country with protracted conflict. Micronutrient deficiencies are highly prevalent among the children of Afghanistan. The prevalence of anemia is 50 percent in children 6 to 24 months old and 38 percent in U5 children. Although lower than those observed in other South Asian countries, these levels are high and warrant urgent attention. Iron and iodine deficiencies both affect 72 percent of U5 children. Scurvy (clinical vitamin C deficiency) has been reported in up to 10 percent of households in some remote, mountainous provinces (Cheung and others 2003).

As figure 1.1 illustrates, the critical window for nutrition intervention is prepregnancy up to 24 months of age (Shrimpton and others 2001). There is consensus that damage to physical growth, cognitive development, and human capital during this period is extensive and largely irreversible (World Bank 2006).

### Maternal Undernutrition: A Significant Challenge

As in many South Asian countries, undernutrition in Afghanistan is not confined to infants and young children. It also afflicts many women of reproductive age. Women and children are the most at risk for malnutrition, although other household members can be affected. The 2004 NNS found 21 percent of women between 15 and 49 years of age to have chronic energy deficiency (body mass index less than 18.5) and 75 percent to have iodine deficiency. The prevalence of iron deficiency and anemia among nonpregnant women in that age group was 48 percent and 25 percent, respectively. The maternal mortality rate (MMR) is fourth highest in the world at 1,600 per 100,000 live births annually, indicating the need for interventions such as early childhood nutrition for girls and improved maternal nutrition (UNICEF 2005). The MMR ranges from

**Figure 1.1    Critical Window of Opportunity for Action: Prepregnancy to 24 Months**

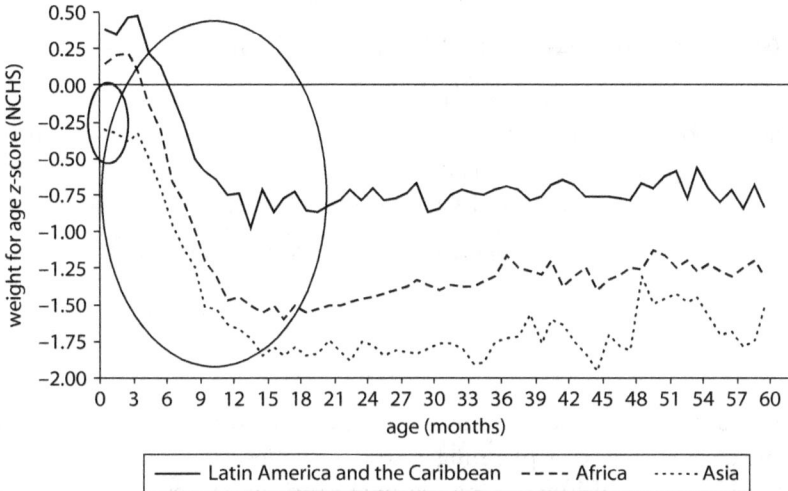

*Source:* World Bank 2006.
*Note:* NCHS = National Center for Health Statistics.

400 per 100,000 live births in Kabul province to 6,500 per 100,000 in Badakhshan province—the highest ever noted globally.

### An Evolving Nutrition Investment Framework

This situation analysis of nutrition in Afghanistan occurs in the context of broader movements within the international development community. During 2009, following a series of high-level meetings, a Global Action Plan (GAP) for Nutrition began to take shape, partly in response to the 2008 *Lancet* series on Maternal and Child Undernutrition. The *Lancet* series identified a host of cost-effective, direct nutrition interventions that could have a significant influence on reducing undernutrition worldwide. Yet the *Lancet* also sounded a call to action because the international nutrition community was deemed "broken ... and lacking leadership" (Horton 2008, 179). The GAP answers this call to action and was informed by a study conducted by the Center for Global Development to understand how and why the international nutrition system is broken and where solutions and renewed leadership might be found (Levine and Kuczynski 2009). Ultimately, the goal of this multipronged movement among concerned stakeholders is to improve international and national infrastructures to support effective, scaled-up nutrition interventions in developing countries (box 1.1). This plan is not prescriptive but rather

**Box 1.1**

## Goal of the Global Action Plan for Nutrition

"The primary objective of the Global Action Plan for Nutrition . . . is to create a global movement and a coordinated and compelling call for action to convince country leaders to scale up nutrition investments to complement ongoing efforts at health systems strengthening, social safety nets, food security, and agriculture."

—Global Action Plan for Nutrition Working Group, 2009

*Source:* "Scaling Up Nutrition (SUN): A Framework for Action."

provides a framework and costed menu of proven interventions that countries can use as a planning resource. It describes the components required for a well-functioning national nutrition system. The GAP has now evolved into the SUN (Scaling Up Nutrition) initiative and has been adopted by more than 80 institutions. The SUN initiative is based on many of the principles and goals in the GAP. This report was written during the period preceding SUN.

The core pillars of the GAP methodology emphasized the following:

• *Pillar 1:* Nutrition is recognized as foundational to national development.
• *Pillar 2:* Adequate local capacity is built and supported to design and execute effective nutrition policies and programs.
• *Pillar 3:* Cost-effective, direct nutrition interventions are scaled up, where applicable.
• *Pillar 4:* Determinants of undernutrition are addressed through multisectoral approaches.
• *Pillar 5:* Coordinated support for nutrition is provided by development partners (including funding for advocacy, communications, and research).

This report examines each of these pillars in the context of Afghanistan. For Pillar 1, the political support for nutrition is examined, as well as the degree to which nutrition is positioned prominently in the development agenda. Institutional and implementation arrangements for nutrition are discussed. Pillar 2 follows on the first, guiding an assessment of local capacity in the government structures primarily responsible for nutrition policies and programs. For Pillar 3, Afghanistan's progress at scaling up direct nutrition interventions that are identified as cost-effective is described. Every country context differs, and each country will need to determine its own set of interventions. Pillar 4 is addressed in two chapters, one relating to an explanation of underlying determinants of nutrition problems (chapter 3) and the other describing the corresponding interventions and gaps in the response (chapter 5). The support and interaction among development partners for advancing nutrition are the focus of Pillar 5.

## Afghanistan: Country Context

Afghanistan has a population of approximately 25 million, with 74 percent living in rural areas (CSO 2009). About half of the population (49 percent) is under age 15 (12 million children), and the total fertility rate is very high at 6.3 children per woman.

Since 1978, ongoing war and internal conflict have displaced millions from their home communities internally or as refugees across international borders. This situation has contributed to ethnic tensions, has resulted in the destruction of infrastructure, and has disrupted government systems. The government established in the post-Taliban period has worked to regain control of the country, restore rural livelihoods, and establish stable governance structures. Education and health care systems, among others, have been revived and are being expanded from urban centers to rural areas.

Afghanistan is home to many tribal ethnic groups, each with their own cultures and traditions. These groups include Pashtuns (42 percent), Tajiks (27 percent), Hazaras (9 percent), Uzbeks (9 percent), Aimaqs (4 percent), Turkmen (3 percent), and Baluchs (2 percent), with the remaining 4 percent from a combination of smaller groups (Girardet and Walter 2004). Though diverse, most of the Afghan population shares a common religion (Islam), a turbulent history, and a language (Pashto or Persian). Most are Muslims: 84 percent are Sunni and 15 percent are Shi'a (primarily the Hazara people).

Afghanistan's culture maintains strong gender roles. Numerous social barriers prevent women from traveling outside the home or working with or providing training to men, although in the cities this trend is changing. Within the household, women are chiefly responsible for child care. However, they have limited influence over how resources are spent and what foods are purchased; men largely make these decisions. Strong gender roles make it more challenging to reach women and children with nutrition messages and services.

The high-risk security environment in large areas of Afghanistan also limits the quality of data collection. Implementing partners have more difficulty providing services (for example, attendance at clinics or health posts), and monitoring is more complicated.

According to the United Nations Refugee Agency, at least 5 million refugees have returned to Afghanistan since 2002, but resuming normal life has been complicated by droughts and the effects of war (UNHCR 2010). Families frequently face land tenure disputes and the destruction of homes, orchards, irrigation systems, and infrastructure because of the bombing, landmines, and "scorched earth" policies of many armies (Girardet and Walter 2004). Poor households have limited stocks of skills and education, thereby constraining their access to profitable diversification as a risk reduction strategy (Pain 2007). Consequently, many poor rural households have moved into livelihoods with low entry costs, such as firewood collection and casual urban or agricultural employment. Households with greater capacities, including stronger social networks, have been better able to meet the entry requirements of shopkeeping, livestock rearing, trade, and migration. One survey of rural households in eight provinces showed that 83 percent obtained some form of wage income, with a mean of US$85 per month and a maximum wage income of US$1,060 per month (Roe 2008). A frequency distribution analysis of these data revealed that 40 percent of households had mean off-farm income of US$42 per month. Households with family members working abroad, in regional centers, or in small businesses were on the higher end of the income spectrum.

The country boasts a dramatic and varied topography, with thousands of microclimates and microwatersheds, leading to changing conditions from one valley to the next and even within valleys on differing slopes (Fitzherbert 2007). Afghanistan's topography is largely mountainous, with the Hindu Kush mountain range covering nearly two-thirds of the country. Most Afghans live in mountain valleys or the plains in the north and southwest. Many areas are inaccessible in winter for aid, markets (such as those for fortified foods), and social services (such as health care). Underlying environmental conditions further affect agriculture, water quality, and livelihood opportunities. This reality underscores the need for localized development planning. The World Bank–supported National Solidarity Program (NSP), which is housed in the Ministry of Rural Rehabilitation and Development (MRRD), is designed to address this need. More than 22,000 NSP community development committees (CDCs) exist and are aided by nongovernment organizations in proposal writing for block grants through MRRD. Another 9,000 CDCs are planned to complete coverage of the country.

According to the Food and Agriculture Organization of the United Nations, only 12 percent of the country (approximately 8 million hectares) is arable. Only 2 percent of the land has remained forested because wood and timber were cut for fuel during the war years. This deforestation has led to extensive desertification, soil erosion, and dust storms. Rivers, underground water sources, snow melts, and rain provide water for livelihood activities and community life. The climate is arid to semi-arid, with cold winters and hot summers. The semi-arid climate poses significant challenges to agricultural production yet benefits soil quality because fewer nutrients are lost to water runoff and plant uptake. A severe drought occurred from 1999 to 2003 that forced many people to abandon agricultural activities and seek alternative employment. Long-term average annual rainfall ranges from 98 millimeters in the south to 579 millimeters in the northeast, with most provinces receiving less than 300 millimeters—below the level needed for crop cultivation (MRRD 2004).

In the midst of a harsh environment, Afghanistan produces an extraordinary range of food and nonfood agricultural products. After decades of conflict, Afghan agriculture had reestablished itself such that in 1997 the country met 70 percent of its food needs through domestic production (Sloane 2001). Over the past three decades, Afghan farmers have become increasingly dynamic, adaptable, and mobile as a population that has been "thrust into the heart of the international market economy" (Fitzherbert 2007, 30). Although Afghan farmers have lost their place in niche markets for dried fruit, nuts, and industrial crops (such as cotton and sugar beet), the export market in mung beans, other pulses, and cumin is growing. Mechanization has expanded, and farmers have improved access to chemical fertilizers in even the remotest rural markets (Fitzherbert 2007). The Afghan government has prioritized horticulture and livestock for investment to offset poppy production. The demand for Afghan higher-value fruits and nuts (as compared to wheat) is great in the nearby Indian market and elsewhere in the region.

Integrated systems of livestock husbandry have coexisted with cropping in a largely symbiotic relationship between pastoralists and settled farmers. In the 1970s, Afghanistan had an estimated 2 million nomadic herders (*Kuchis*), but drought, deteriorating rangeland, and livestock losses have reduced their numbers to only a few tens of thousands (Fitzherbert 2007). The reduced livestock population has also compromised the availability and affordability of animal-source foods at the household level and in area markets (MRRD 2004). Data from 2003 surveys at sentinel sites around the country found that a greater percentage of households consumed animal-source foods if they owned the corresponding asset ($p < 0.001$) (Johnecheck and Holland 2005).

## Methods and Analytical Approach

The methods used in the compilation of this report included

- Network assessment of key stakeholders in nutrition in Afghanistan
- Analysis of available nutritional epidemiology data
- Analysis of available knowledge-attitudes-practices data
- Review of the MOPH Basic Package of Health Services (BPHS) regarding nutrition
- Review of programs in nonhealth sectors that affect or could affect nutrition
- Capacity assessment of the MOPH Public Nutrition Department and other nutrition-relevant institutional structures to lead and implement scaled-up, effective multisectoral nutrition interventions

The analytical approach was based on the nutrition investment framework provided by the Global Action Plan for Nutrition. The interpretation of the data is structured according to the five pillars deemed to be necessary for progress in reducing undernutrition at the country level. A complete presentation of methods is found in appendix A, and interviews conducted are listed in appendix B.

## Structure of the Report

The report is organized into six chapters. Chapter 2 gives an overview of the nutrition situation in Afghanistan, focusing particularly on the following topics: child undernutrition, maternal undernutrition, and vitamin and mineral deficiencies. Chapter 3 presents the United Nations Children's Fund (UNICEF) framework used to explore underlying determinants of nutrition problems in Afghanistan. The UNICEF framework is applied through a systematic description of key factors underlying malnutrition, including food security, health and health services, health environment, care for women and children, and nutrition awareness. Chapter 4 reviews Afghanistan's nutrition infrastructure and institutional arrangements to support nutrition policies and programs. Chapter 5 covers the program efforts, gaps, and opportunities facing the Afghan government and its partners working in nutrition. Finally, chapter 6 makes a series of policy and programmatic recommendations to elucidate next steps for address-ing the identified gaps and challenges to improved nutrition for the Afghan population.

## Note

1. The basic idea of the Copenhagen Consensus is to bring a group of the world's leading economists together to answer this question: "Imagine you had US\$75 billion to donate to worthwhile causes. What would you do, and where should we start?" The exercise is carried out every four years to ensure that new, important challenges and solutions are included in the process and that research is updated.

## References

Cheung, Edith, Roya Mutahar, Fitsum Assefa, Mija-Tesse Ververs, Shah Mahmood Nasiri, Annalies Borrel, and Peter Salama. 2003. "An Epidemic of Scurvy in Afghanistan: Assessment and Response." *Food and Nutrition Bulletin* 24 (3): 247–55.

CSO (Central Statistics Office). 2009. *National Risk and Vulnerability Assessment 2007/08: A Profile of Afghanistan.* Kabul: Ministry of Rural Rehabilitation and Development.

Fitzherbert, Anthony. 2007. "Rural Resilience and Diversity across Afghanistan's Agricultural Landscapes." In *Reconstructing Agriculture in Afghanistan*, ed. Adam Pain and Jacky Sutton, 29–48. Warwickshire, U.K.: United Nations Food and Agriculture Organization.

Girardet, Edward, and Jonathan Walter. 2004. *Afghanistan*. 2nd ed. Geneva: Media Action International.

Horton, Richard. 2008. "Maternal and Child Undernutrition: An Urgent Opportunity." *Lancet* 371 (9608): 179.

Johnecheck, Wendy, and Diane Holland. 2005. "Nutritional Risk in Afghanistan: Evidence from the NSS Pilot Study (2003–2004) and the NRVA 2003." Tufts University, Medford, MA.

Levine, Ruth, and Danielle Kuczynski. 2009. "Review of the Global Nutrition Landscape." Center for Global Development, Washington, DC.

MOPH (Ministry of Public Health). 2009. "Strategy on Prevention and Control of Vitamin and Mineral Deficiencies in Afghanistan." Public Nutrition Department, MOPH, Kabul.

MOPH (Ministry of Public Health), UNICEF (United Nations Children's Fund), CDC (Centers for Disease Control and Prevention), National Institute for Research on Food and Nutrition–Italy, and Tufts University. 2009. *2004 Afghanistan National Nutrition Survey.* Atlanta: CDC.

MRRD (Ministry of Rural Rehabilitation and Development). 2004. "Analysis of Drought Impact in Afghanistan." MRRD, Kabul.

Pain, Adam. 2007. "Rural Livelihoods in Afghanistan." In *Reconstructing Agriculture in Afghanistan,* ed. Adam Pain and Jacky Sutton, 49–64. Warwickshire, U.K.: United Nations Food and Agriculture Organization.

Pinstrup-Andersen, Per, and Satoru Shimokawa. 2008. "Do Poverty and Poor Health and Nutrition Increase the Risk of Armed Conflict Onset?" *Food Policy* 33 (6): 513–20.

Roe, Alan, 2008. *Water Management, Livestock, and the Opium Economy: Natural Resources Management, Farming Systems, and Rural Livelihoods.* Kabul: Afghanistan Research and Evaluation Unit.

Shrimpton, Roger, Cesar G. Victora, Mercedes de Onis, Rosângela Costa Lima, Monika Blössner, and Graeme Clugston. 2001. "The Worldwide Timing of Growth Faltering: Implications for Nutritional Interventions." *Pediatrics* 107 (5): e75.

Sloane, Peter. 2001. "Food Security for Afghanistan." Revised version of a paper presented at the International Conference on Analytical Foundations for Assistance to Afghanistan held by the United Nations Development Programme and World Bank, Islamabad, June 5–6.

UNHCR (United Nations Refugee Agency). 2010. "2010 UNHCR Country Operations Profile: Afghanistan." UNCHR, Geneva. http://www.unhcr.org/cgi-bin/texis/vtx/page?page=49e486eb6.

UNICEF (United Nations Children's Fund). 2005. "Afghanistan Country Statistics." UNICEF, New York. http://www.unicef.org/infobycountry/afghanistan_statistics.html.

World Bank. 2006. *Repositioning Nutrition as Central to Development: A Strategy for Large-Scale Action.* Washington, DC: World Bank.

# CHAPTER 2

# The Current Nutrition Situation in Afghanistan

Data on child and maternal undernutrition were obtained from the 2004 National Nutrition Survey (NNS) (MOPH and others 2009), which is the only comprehensive national nutrition study of its kind for the country. With support from the U.S. Centers for Disease Control and Prevention, the summary data, using National Center for Health Statistics (NCHS) references, were released in 2005. In late 2009, a detailed NNS report was published, using instead the updated World Health Organization (WHO) growth references. Appendix B contains a summary of all identified nutrition-related data sources. Because of the cluster sampling methodology, NNS data cannot be used for provincial-level estimates. Of the 39 clusters in the design, 32 provided adequate data for analysis. Age and gender breakdowns are available for each undernutrition condition. Mother's and father's education level and literacy are used as proxies for socioeconomic status and are used only with that individual's nutrition indicators. Parental education represents the only measure of socioeconomic status in the NNS. Geographic disaggregation is available only for iodized salt consumption, presented as Kabul compared with other clusters. These data largely confirm regional reports that were compiled to write the first iteration of the National Public Nutrition Policy and Strategy (2003–06). The policy was updated with these national figures in 2005. These NNS figures continue to be used for national planning in nutrition. Data on underlying causes (for example, child feeding, food security, and access to safe drinking water) are updated more frequently through other national surveys.

## Child Undernutrition: Overview

Definitions of relevant nutrition terms are found in the glossary.

According to WHO classifications, growth stunting and underweight are of "very high" public health significance in Afghanistan for children under five years of age (U5). Wasting is of "medium" severity for U5 children. Gender differences were not identified for any form of child undernutrition in the NNS. Table 2.1 shows the WHO classification for degree of public health significance for growth stunting, underweight, and wasting among U5 children.

### *Growth Stunting*

Childhood growth stunting represents a priority challenge for national development. Growth stunting adversely affects children, regardless of gender, through decreased motor and cognitive development as well as lifetime work capacity. For girls, it may lead to obstructed labor caused by small hips later in life. This condition and postpartum hemorrhage, which is related to obstructed labor, are the leading causes of the extremely high maternal mortality in Afghanistan (Bartlett and others 2002; Ververs 2005). Early age of marriage and pregnancy further retard optimal growth of young mothers.

**Table 2.1    Public Health Significance of Child Undernutrition in Afghanistan**

| | Prevalence (%) | | | |
|---|---|---|---|---|
| *Undernutrition characteristic* | *Low* | *Medium* | *High* | *Very high* |
| *WHO classification (global)* | | | | |
| Stunting | < 20 | 20–29 | 30–39 | ≥ 40 |
| Underweight | < 10 | 10–19 | 20–29 | ≥ 30 |
| Wasting | < 5 | 5–9 | 10–14 | ≥ 15 |
| *Afghanistan 2004 NNS: all children 6.0–59.9 months* | | | | |
| Stunting | | | | 60.5 |
| Underweight | | | | 33.7 |
| Wasting | | 8.7 | | |

*Source:* WHO 1995.
*Note:* Data for Afghanistan show where Afghanistan falls within the WHO classification.

Growth stunting is a very serious problem in Afghanistan and occurs in three of five U5 children (60.5 percent).[1] Boys (61.2 percent) and girls (59.6 percent) showed no significant difference. Among children under two years of age (U2), 41.9 percent of children 6.0 to 11.9 months old already showed stunted growth, as did 53.4 percent of those 12.0 to 23.9 months old (figure 2.1). This finding indicates the early onset of the problem and the critical nature of proper feeding, hygiene, health, and care practices in the first two years of life.

## Underweight

The prevalence of underweight was 33.7 percent in U5 children.[2] No differences were found on the basis of gender (32.9 percent of boys, 34.7 percent of girls). For children 6.0 to 11.9 months old, 29.8 percent were underweight, and for those 12.0 to 23.9 months old, 34.7 percent (figure 2.1). Up to a third of child mortality is attributable to the synergistic effect of undernutrition (underweight) and infection (Black and others 2008). With high mortality rates for infants (111 per 1,000 live births) and U5 children (161 per 1,000), the government of Afghanistan and its development partners must act swiftly to ensure child survival and the ability of future generations to achieve their full physical and intellectual potential (CSO 2009).

**Figure 2.1    Child Undernutrition by Age Group, from the 2004 NNS**

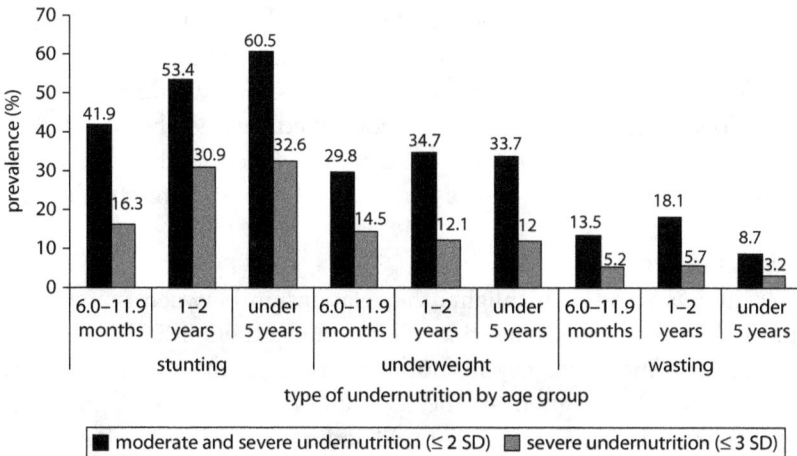

Source: MOPH and others 2009, using the WHO growth references.
Note: SD = standard deviations.

## Wasting

Global acute malnutrition (undernutrition) was 8.7 percent in U5 children.[3] There were no significant differences by gender (boys 8.0 percent, girls 9.4 percent). The highest prevalence by age grouping occurred among children one to two years old (18.1 percent). Children 6.0 to 11.9 months old had a prevalence of 13.5 percent (figure 2.1). The result for U5 children is surprising because Afghanistan has been in a state of chronic conflict since the late 1970s, which would lead to expectations of higher levels of wasting (for example, the Democratic Republic of Congo has wasting levels ranging from 20 to 30 percent depending on the province). The present data provide evidence of a need for a longer-term response to undernutrition in Afghanistan to complement a shorter-term, emergency-oriented response. The one- to two-year age group most affected merits additional examination to determine why the rates are highest during this period. Wasting is caused by inadequate food intake. Possible explanations include sudden or abrupt weaning attributable to successive pregnancy (a common practice in Afghanistan), short birth intervals, slow transition to the family diet, and higher rates of illness (and loss of appetite) as the child becomes more mobile. Chapter 3 provides relevant information on underlying causes.

## Child Undernutrition: Vitamin and Mineral Deficiencies

The 2004 NNS provides the first-ever countrywide data on the micronutrient status of the Afghan population. Iodine and iron data were collected from 15 less geographically remote clusters (of the usable 32 clusters sampled); these data are believed to be underestimates because these clusters provided greater access to markets and services than would more remote areas. No significant differences were identified between boys and girls in prevalence of any of the vitamin or mineral deficiencies, but some differences were seen by age. Data are summarized for children in table 2.2.

## Iodine Deficiency

A recent *Lancet* series highlights the relationship between maternal and child iodine deficiency conditions (Black and others 2008). Even mild, subclinical iodine deficiency in mothers during pregnancy impairs motor and cognitive development of the fetus and increases risk of miscarriage and fetal growth restriction. Breast milk iodine content is very low in areas of endemic iodine deficiency (such as Afghanistan), worsening depletion in infants and increasing risk of developmental problems. Iodine deficiency

**Table 2.2    Vitamin and Mineral Deficiencies among Afghan Preschool Children**

| Deficiency | Preschool children, 6–59 months (%) |
|---|---|
| Iodine deficiency (urinary iodine < 100 μg/L) | 71.9[a] |
| Iron deficiency (zinc protoporphyrin) | 71.5 |
| Anemia (hemoglobin 11 g/dL) | 37.9 (50 in 6–24 months) |
| Iron-deficiency anemia (hemoglobin and zinc protoporphyrin) | 33.4 (55 in 12–24 months) |
| Zinc deficiency (estimated from stunting and iron deficiency) | 54–72[b] |
| Vitamin A deficiency (from serum retinol) | 28[c] |

*Source:* MOPH and others 2009, except where noted.
a. No data for U5 children. Figure estimated from the prevalence of iodine deficiency in school-age children.
b. Black and others (2008) recommends estimating zinc deficiency in U5 children from the stunting estimate and measures of zinc bioavailability in the food supply. Some authors have come up with figures less than 20 percent. This result seems unlikely given iron-deficiency levels. Zinc-deficiency levels often are similar to iron-deficiency levels.
c. Problems occurred with the transport of serum retinol samples in the 2004 NNS. Vitamin A data for children are measured using serum retinol concentrations from blood samples in a subsample of 47 children in Kabul.

is the main cause of preventable mental retardation around the world. Populations with chronic iodine deficiency have an average of 13 IQ points lower than iodine-sufficient populations (Zimmermann, Jooste, and Pandav 2008).

Iodine deficiency data were collected only for women and school-age children. No data exist for U5 children. However, the data on school-age children (7–12 years of age) are taken to be a proxy for levels in younger children. Prevalence of iodine deficiency in school-age children was 71.9 percent (69.9 percent boys, 73.4 percent girls), with a higher prevalence of iodine deficiency in clusters outside of Kabul (see figure 2.2).

### Iron Deficiency and Anemia

Iron-deficient women may give birth to infants with reduced iron stores. Infants with low iron stores may become anemic as early as three months of age, whereas healthy infants usually have stores lasting as long as six months (Yip and Dallman 1996). Iron-deficiency anemia can irreparably damage children's cognitive development if deficiencies occur during the first two years of life (WHO 2001). Iron-deficiency anemia is also associated with poor growth (Rivera and others 2003).

The 2004 NNS found that 71.5 percent of children 6 to 59 months old (U5) had iron deficiency. A similar proportion of boys (70.1 percent) and girls (72.9 percent) were deficient. Almost all children 6 to 12 months

**Figure 2.2    Proportion of Iodine-Deficient Nonpregnant Women and School-Age Children in Kabul Compared with the Rest of the Country**

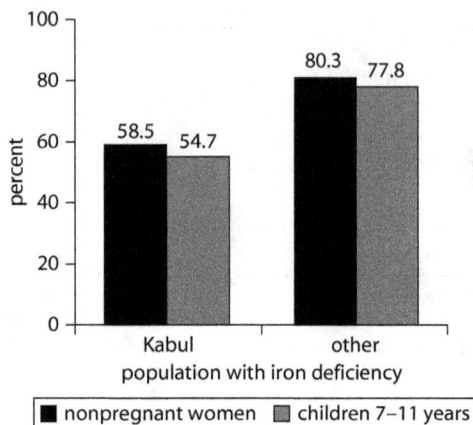

*Source:* MOPH and others 2009.

old were deficient (96.2 percent). Because breast milk is low in iron, iron-rich foods are critical after six months of age, when iron stores from gestation are exhausted. Furthermore, iron-rich food is critical in preventing and managing infections (for example, diarrhea) to reduce iron losses. The lowest prevalence was among four- to five-year-olds (51.9 percent). Approximately half of those with iron deficiency (38 percent) had anemia (hemoglobin less than 11 grams per deciliter). There were no significant differences by gender (37.2 percent males, 38.6 percent females). Half (49.7 percent) of those 6 to 24 months old had anemia, and children 12 to 24 months had the highest prevalence (59.6 percent). Table 2.3 illustrates anemia differences by age group.

## Zinc Deficiency

A recent review of the effects of zinc deficiency is provided in the 2008 *Lancet* series on maternal and child undernutrition (Black and others 2008). Zinc deficiency results in an increased risk of pneumonia, malaria, and diarrhea in areas where these diseases are present. A lack of zinc further affects the frequency and severity of diarrhea, a leading cause of child death in Afghanistan. Approximately 4 percent of deaths in U5 children are attributable to zinc deficiency. Treatment of diarrhea with oral rehydration solution in parallel with a zinc supplement regimen for 10 to 14 days provides greater recovery to children and reduces school days lost (for older children). Growth stunting is one clinical manifestation of zinc

**Table 2.3    Prevalence of Anemia among U5 Children**

| Age group (months)* | Anemia[a] (%) | Mean hemoglobin (g/dL) |
|---|---|---|
| 6–11.9 | 33.1 | 11.3 |
| 12–23.9 | 59.6 | 10.4 |
| 24–35.9 | 49.0 | 10.9 |
| 36–47.9 | 36.5 | 11.3 |
| 48–59.9 | 17.5 | 11.8 |
| National | 37.9 | 11.2 |

Source: MOPH and others 2009.
a. Anemia cutoff for preschool children is hemoglobin (Hb) < 11.0 grams/deciliter. Hb is measured by HemoCue and adjusted for altitude.
* $p < 0.05$

deficiency, and supplementation has been shown to have a direct positive effect on improving linear growth (Brown and others 2002). On a routine basis, children need not only zinc supplements when they suffer from diarrhea, but also regular consumption of zinc-rich foods (typically foods that are fortified). Fortified complementary foods and home-level fortification using micronutrient powders are avenues being explored globally for addressing zinc deficiency (Martorell 2002).

No direct data on zinc deficiency are available for Afghanistan; however, estimates of zinc deficiency are taken from the U5 children stunting statistic of 60.5 percent. Where possible, this estimate is combined with the adequacy of absorbable zinc in the country's food supply. Other estimates for zinc deficiency are sometimes made using iron-deficiency rates, because both deficiencies often occur together, given the similar food sources of these nutrients. If zinc deficiency were estimated on the basis of the iron-deficiency rate in Afghanistan, prevalence in children would be above 70 percent. The revised Basic Package of Health Services (BPHS) now includes zinc supplementation with oral rehydration solution for diarrhea treatment although it is not yet at scale.

### Vitamin A Deficiency

Vitamin A deficiency (VAD) contributes significantly to child mortality, poor eye health, and blindness. Vitamin A supplementation has been shown to reduce child mortality by 23 percent on average (Bhutta and others 2008).

Although Afghanistan has no national-level biological measures of VAD, it is expected to be high for various reasons. The only available data from the 2004 NNS pertain to maternal night blindness. Where night blindness during pregnancy is prevalent, xerophthalmia (corneal degeneration) tends to be highly prevalent in children. The prevalence of VAD among children is likely to be high in this population, given that maternal night blindness was recorded at 10 percent (MOPH and others 2009).[4] Although children's serum samples were generally unavailable, prevalence was measured on a subsample of (only) 47 U5 children from Kabul, 13 of whom (28 percent) showed VAD (MOPH and others 2009). Because access to services and food security may be worse in more remote, rural areas, this figure is viewed as an underestimate of the prevalence of VAD in Afghan children. These children were not significantly different from other children in the NNS in terms of age, sex, wasting, low weight for age, or anemia. The very high incidence of infant and child mortality and morbidity also suggests more widespread VAD. The high coverage of vitamin A supplements (more than 90 percent according to recent MOPH estimates) temporarily treats the deficiency in children's diets. Chapter 3 provides more details on supplementation activities.

### Vitamin C Deficiency

Vitamin C deficiency (scurvy) was documented in 10 percent of the population in some remote, mountainous provinces during surveys in 2003 (Cheung and others 2003). Reports of scurvy have decreased, yet this decrease may only be because of emergency-oriented interventions supported by the United Nations Children's Fund for at-risk areas (for example, Ghor province) to avert outbreaks during the long winter months.

### Vitamin D Deficiency

Prevalence of vitamin D deficiency (for example, rickets) is unknown in Afghanistan, but pilot studies indicated a significant population deficiency (MOPH and others 2009). Vitamin D is important for bone health because it helps in calcium absorption. Humans can synthesize vitamin D from sunlight exposure, but conservative dress customs and extreme weather in Afghanistan may complicate such synthesis. A vitamin D study is under way in Badakhshan, Baghlan, and Bamyan provinces with sponsorship from the Aga Khan Development Network.[5]

## Maternal Undernutrition: Underweight

Maternal underweight poses a problem for the woman's own health and for the intergenerational cycle of undernutrition. Underweight mothers are more likely to have infants with low birth weight (LBW). LBW children born are at increased risk of dying, and those who survive grow at reduced rates throughout their lives. Evidence also links higher incidence of nutrition-related chronic diseases later in life with LBW and growth-stunted children (Victora and others 2008).

Among nonpregnant women, 20.9 percent had a body mass index (BMI) below 18.5 (weight divided by height squared, expressed as kilograms per square meter), indicating chronic energy deficiency. This percentage is viewed as an underestimate, because women were weighed while wearing clothing. According to the WHO standards (1995), prevalence of chronic energy deficiency above 20 percent is considered high and a serious public health problem (table 2.4).

## School-Age Children and Adults: Vitamin and Mineral Deficiencies

Among school-age children, only iodine-deficiency data were collected. For adults, major differences occurred among males and females in micronutrient status (see table 2.5). Differences were also identified in some adults by education level.

### Iodine Deficiency

Consequences of iodine deficiency have largely been discussed in this chapter. Iodine deficiency can cause birth defects such as cretinism and mental retardation if the mother is deficient, as well as goiter. At least three-quarters of women (74.7 percent nonpregnant, 78.9 percent pregnant) had iodine deficiency (see table 2.5). Among nonpregnant women, those with at minimum a primary education were less likely to be deficient (54.5 percent) than were those without any formal schooling (77.0 percent). School-age children (7–11 years) also had high levels of iodine deficiency, averaging 71.9 percent. No data were collected for

**Table 2.4    The Public Health Significance of Different Ranges of Prevalence of Low BMI among Nonpregnant Women 15 to 49 Years Old[a]**

| | | Prevalence (%) | | |
|---|---|---|---|---|
| Normal | Low (warning sign, monitoring required) | Medium (poor situation) | High (serious situation) | Very high (critical situation) |
| 3–5 | 5–9 | 10–19 | 20–39 **(20.1 BMI)[b]** | ≥ 40 |

*Source:* WHO 1995.
a. Low BMI is defined as 18.5 kg/mg$^2$.
b. Afghanistan's prevalence is high.

**Table 2.5    Vitamin and Mineral Deficiencies for School-Age Children and Adults**

| | Prevalence (%) | | | |
| --- | --- | --- | --- | --- |
| Deficiency | School-age children (7–11 years) | Nonpregnant women (15–49 years) | Pregnant women (15–49 years) | Men (18–60 years) |
| Iodine deficiency (urinary iodine < 100 μg/L) | 71.9 | 74.7 | 78.9 | — |
| Iron deficiency (zinc protoporphyrin) | — | 48.4 | 65.3 | 18.0 |
| Anemia[a] (hemoglobin) | — | 24.7 | 25.7 | 7.1 |
| Iron-deficiency anemia (hemoglobin and zinc protoporphyrin) | — | 15.8 | 25.0 | 4.2 |
| Zinc deficiency[b] | — | 48 | 65 | 18 |
| Vitamin A deficiency (night blindness as proxy) | — | — | 9.9–20.0[c] | — |
| Vitamin C deficiency (scurvy; bleeding gums[d] as proxy) | Up to 10 in certain regions | | | |

*Source:* MOPH and others 2009, except where noted.

Note: — = not available.

a. Hemoglobin (Hb) is adjusted for altitude and cigarette smoking (men only). Anemia was defined as Hb less than 11.0 grams/deciliter (g/dL) for pregnant women, Hb < 12.0 g/dL for nonpregnant women, and Hb < 13.0 g/dL for men.

b. Estimated from iron deficiency prevalence because no data currently exist on zinc deficiency for this population and these two deficiencies typically occur together.

c. Maternal VAD is measured using the symptom of night blindness. The 2004 NNS recorded 9.9 percent of pregnant women as having night blindness. A meta-analysis of regional nongovernment organization surveys found a mean of 20.0 percent night blindness (Dufour and Borrel 2007).

d. Data are from Cheung and others (2003).

men. The deficiency was greater in clusters outside Kabul than within Kabul (figure 2.2).

## Iron Deficiency and Anemia

Because of the critical role of iron in energy metabolism, insufficient iron affects productivity in adults even for those performing relatively light work (Horton and Ross 2003). Among nonpregnant women, 48.4 percent had iron deficiency, and 24.7 percent had anemia. Of pregnant women, 65.3 percent had iron deficiency, and 25.7 percent had anemia. Younger age, illiteracy, and less education were significantly associated with prevalence of iron deficiency and anemia in nonpregnant women (table 2.6). The presence of few educated pregnant women prevented further analysis by education in this group.

For women, postpartum hemorrhage is one of the two leading causes of maternal death in Afghanistan (Ververs 2005). Anemic mothers have

**Table 2.6    Prevalence of Women with Anemia, Based on Pregnancy Status and Educational Characteristics**

| Characteristics of women (15–49 years) | Pregnant women | | Nonpregnant women | |
|---|---|---|---|---|
| | Anemia (%) | Mean hemoglobin (g/dL) | Anemia (%) | Mean hemoglobin (g/dL) |
| *Literacy* | | | | |
| Illiterate | 26.0 | 12.8 | 27.0* | 12.8 |
| Can read | 19.2 | 12.7 | 7.1* | 13.2 |
| *Education* | | | | |
| No school | 25.0 | 12.8 | 27.0* | 12.8 |
| Primary or secondary school | 20.2 | 12.6 | 7.3* | 13.1 |
| High school or higher | — | — | — | — |
| National | 24.7 | 12.8 | 25.7 | 12.9 |

*Source:* MOPH and others 2009.
*Note:* — = not available. Weighted analysis for prevalence to account for complex survey design. Anemia cutoff for nonpregnant and pregnant women is hemoglobin (Hb) < 12.0 g/dL and Hb < 11.0 g/dL, respectively. Hb is measured by HemoCue and adjusted for altitude and pregnancy status. Means are weighted and standard deviations are calculated assuming simple random sampling.
*p < 0.05 difference between pregnant and nonpregnant women.

a higher mortality than nonanemic mothers; a 1 gram per deciliter increase in hemoglobin status (between 5 and 12 grams per deciliter) translates to a 20 percent decrease in mortality risk according to the WHO. Compounded by VAD and chronic energy deficiency, anemia has important implications for child care and income-earning activities (Dreyfuss and others 2000).

For men (18–60 years), 18.0 percent had iron deficiency and 7.1 percent had anemia. Literate men were less likely to be iron deficient. Men who were literate and more educated were less likely to be anemic.

### Zinc Deficiency

Zinc deficiency in adults causes a range of health problems, including increased morbidity risk. Although no data exist on zinc deficiency for the population, estimates can be made from iron-deficiency rates because both deficiencies often occur together. If such is the case in Afghanistan, prevalence in nonpregnant women would be near 50 percent and in men, 18 percent.

### Vitamin A Deficiency

In women, VAD causes night blindness, particularly during pregnancy. Serum retinol estimates are unavailable for the population because of problems transporting laboratory samples during the 2004 NNS. Almost

10 percent of pregnant women self-reported night blindness, and this figure is believed to be an underestimate. Earlier data from varied non-government organization surveys consistently found approximately 20 percent of women having night blindness (Dufour and Borrel 2007). A maternal night blindness prevalence equal to or greater than 5 percent indicates a community VAD problem that is of public health significance (Christian 2002).

### Folic Acid (Folate) Deficiency (Vitamin B$_9$)

Folate enables the healthy development of the central nervous system and is essential in the development of new cells. In the first few weeks of pregnancy, low folate intake leads to infants being born with neural tube defects such as spina bifida and anencephaly (Wald and others 2001). Folate deficiency can also cause anemia.

Data on birth outcomes from Rabia Balkhi Hospital in Kabul report an incidence of spina bifida and anencephaly of 60 per 10,000 births (MOPH and others 2009). This rate is almost eight times that in Canada or the United States and suggests substantial folate deficiency among those mothers. These data come from a major urban hospital, suggesting that the situation is likely worse in remote, rural areas.

### Overweight and Obesity: Children and Women

Data are available for children and women on overweight and obesity. In the 2004 NNS, data show 4.7 percent of children 6 to 59 months old were overweight, having weight-for-height scores more than two standard deviations above the mean. By contrast, 2.3 percent of children in the reference population are overweight. Among U5 boys, the prevalence was 6.6 percent, and among U5 girls, it was 2.4 percent. No significant differences are reported by gender. The highest levels were found in children 3 to 4 years (6.0 percent) and 4 to 5 years (6.8 percent).

In the same survey, 12.2 percent of nonpregnant women were overweight (BMI 25.0–29.9), and 3.4 percent were obese (BMI greater than 30).

### Summary of Data and Data Gaps

Three in five of Afghanistan's children are chronically undernourished, and high proportions suffer from vitamin and mineral deficiencies. Nearly all (96.2 percent) children 6 to 12 months old were iron deficient, and 50 percent of those 6 to 24 months old were anemic. Wasting is of lower prevalence than anticipated (8.7 percent), but among children one to two years old, 18 percent were acutely undernourished. Maternal underweight (more than 20 percent) is a problem of serious public health significance. Women also experienced high levels of iodine and iron deficiency, and a quarter of nonpregnant women were anemic. Night blindness levels of 10 percent indicate a problem with VAD in the general population. Appendix B summarizes available national data sources relevant to nutrition.

The data presented in this chapter provide strong justification for action to address maternal and child undernutrition, yet no national data sets permit disaggregated analysis of undernutrition by district or province or by urban versus rural areas or allow cross-tabulation by socioeconomic status indicators. This type of disaggregation would enable better targeting of interventions (for example, selection of higher-priority provinces). In the absence of such data, proxy indicators (for example, U5 mortality, maternal mortality) could be used.

Afghanistan would benefit from a standardized, periodic survey that assessed individual nutritional status (including vitamins and minerals) of the population. These surveys should be designed to enable disaggregated analysis of undernutrition by district or province or by urban versus rural areas or to allow cross-tabulation by socioeconomic status indicators. The disaggregation would facilitate use of data for program planning, and the standardization would enable tracking of trends.

The National Risk and Vulnerability Assessment measures food security indicators only at the household level (see chapter 3). A Multiple Indicator Cluster Survey, which will include nutrition indicators, is planned for spring 2010, sponsored by the United Nations Children's Fund. Specifically, no population-level data are available for iodine deficiency in U5 children, nor do such data exist for zinc deficiency, VAD (apart from night blindness among pregnant women), folate deficiency (particularly women and adolescent girls), vitamin C deficiency, and vitamin D deficiency.

## Notes

1. According to NCHS references, stunting appeared in 54 percent of children under five years of age and 46 percent of children under two years of age, and there were no significant gender differences.

2. According to NCHS references, the prevalence of underweight was 39.3 percent in U5 children and 39.7 percent in U2 children, with no gender differences.

3. According to NCHS references, the wasting prevalence was 6.7 percent in U5 children and 12.6 percent in U2 children, with no gender differences (inclusive of children less than or equal to two and less than or equal to three standard deviations).

4. A maternal night blindness prevalence equal to or greater than 5 percent indicates a community VAD problem and is declared a problem of public health significance (Christian 2002).

5. Personal communication, Dr. Adela Mubasher, WHO Afghanistan.

## References

Bartlett, Linda, Sara Whitehead, Chadd Crouse, Sonya Bowens, Shairose Mawji, Denisa Ionete, and Peter Salama. 2002. "Maternal Mortality in Afghanistan: Magnitude, Causes, Risk Factors, and Preventability." Afghan Ministry of Public Health, U.S. Centers for Disease Control and Prevention, and United Nations Children's Fund, Kabul.

Bhutta, Zulfiqar A., Tahmeed Ahmed, Robert E. Black, Simon Cousens, Kathryn Dewey, Elsa Giugliani, Batool A. Haider, Betty Kirkwood, Saul S. Morris, H. P. S. Sachdev, and Meera Shekar. 2008. "What Works? Interventions for Maternal and Child Undernutrition and Survival." *Lancet* 371 (9608): 417–40.

Black, Robert E., Lindsay H. Allen, Zulfiqar A. Bhutta, Laura E. Caulfield, Mercedes de Onis, Majid Ezzati, Colin Mathers, and Juan Rivera. 2008. "Maternal and Child Undernutrition: Global and Regional Exposures and Health Consequences." *Lancet* 371 (9608): 243–60.

Brown, Kenneth H., Janet M. Peerson, Juan Rivera, and Lindsay H. Allen. 2002. "Effect of Supplemental Zinc on the Growth and Serum Zinc Concentrations of Prepubertal Children: A Meta-analysis of Randomized Controlled Trials." *American Journal of Clinical Nutrition* 75 (6): 1062–71.

Cheung, Edith, Roya Mutahar, Fitsum Assefa, Mija-Tesse Ververs, Shah Mahmood Nasiri, Annalies Borrel, and Peter Salama. 2003. "An Epidemic of Scurvy in Afghanistan: Assessment and Response." *Food and Nutrition Bulletin* 24 (3): 247–55.

Christian, Parul. 2002. "Recommendations for Indicators: Night Blindness during Pregnancy—a Simple Tool to Assess Vitamin A Deficiency in a Population." *Journal of Nutrition* 132 (9 suppl): 2884S–88S.

CSO (Central Statistics Office). 2009. *National Risk and Vulnerability Assessment 2007/08: A Profile of Afghanistan.* Kabul: Ministry of Rural Rehabilitation and Development.

Dreyfuss, Michelle L., Rebecca J. Stoltzfus, Jaya B. Shrestha, Elizabeth K. Pradhan, Steven C. LeClerq, Subarna K. Khatry, Sharada R. Shrestha, Joanne Katz, Marco Albonico, and Keith P. West Jr. 2000. "Hookworms, Malaria, and

Vitamin A Deficiency Contribute to Anemia and Iron Deficiency among Pregnant Women in the Plains of Nepal." *Journal of Nutrition* 130 (10): 2527–36.

Dufour, Charlotte, and Annalies Borrel. 2007. "Towards a Public Nutrition Response in Afghanistan: Evolutions in Nutritional Assessment and Response." In *Reconstructing Agriculture in Afghanistan*, ed. Adam Pain and Jacky Sutton, 93–118. Warwickshire, U.K.: Practical Action.

Horton, Susan, and Jay Ross. 2003. "The Economics of Iron Deficiency." *Food Policy* 28 (1): 51–75.

Martorell, Reynaldo. 2002. "Benefits of Zinc Supplementation for Child Growth." *American Journal of Clinical Nutrition* 75 (6): 957–58.

MOPH (Ministry of Public Health), UNICEF (United Nations Children's Fund), CDC (Centers for Disease Control and Prevention), National Institute for Research on Food and Nutrition–Italy, and Tufts University. 2009. *2004 Afghanistan National Nutrition Survey*. Atlanta: CDC.

Rivera, Juan A., Christine Hotz, Teresa González-Cossío, Lynette Neufeld, and Armando García-Guerra. 2003. "The Effect of Micronutrient Deficiencies on Child Growth: A Review of Results from Community-Based Supplementation Trials." *Journal of Nutrition* 133 (11 suppl 2): 4010S–20S.

Ververs, Mija-Tesse. 2005. "Improving the Nutrition Status of Afghan Women of Reproductive Age: Recommendations towards the Development of a Maternal Nutrition Strategy." United Nations Children's Fund, Kabul.

Victora, Cesar G., Linda Adair, Caroline Fall, Pedro C. Hallal, Reynaldo Martorell, Linda Richter, and Harshpal Singh Sachdev for the Maternal and Child Undernutrition Study Group. 2008. "Maternal and Child Undernutrition: Consequences for Adult Health and Human Capital." *Lancet* 371 (9608): 340–57.

Wald, Nicholas J., Malcolm R. Law, Joan K. Morris, and David S. Wald. 2001. "Quantifying the Effect of Folic Acid." *Lancet* 358 (9298): 2069–73.

WHO (World Health Organization). 1995. *Physical Status: The Use and Interpretation of Anthropometry*. Geneva: WHO.

———. 2001. *Iron Deficiency Anaemia: Assessment, Prevention, and Control—A Guide for Programme Managers*. Geneva: WHO.

Yip, Ray, and Peter R. Dallman. 1996. "Iron." In *Present Knowledge in Nutrition*, 7th ed., ed. Ekhard Ziegler and L. J. Filer Jr., 277–92. Washington, DC: ILSI.

Zimmermann, Michael B., Pieter L. Jooste, and Chandrakant S. Pandav. 2008. "Iodine-Deficiency Disorders." *Lancet* 372 (9645): 1251–62.

# CHAPTER 3

# The Determinants of Undernutrition in Afghanistan

## The UNICEF Framework

The nutrition community in Afghanistan has adopted the United Nations Children's Fund (UNICEF) framework for the causes of undernutrition (figure 3.1) in policy and program documents (UNICEF 1990). In the UNICEF framework, malnutrition—represented in its different forms of undernutrition and overnutrition—is explained as resulting from varying levels of immediate, underlying, and basic causes. Given the relatively low levels of overnutrition in Afghanistan, malnutrition is understood in this assessment as undernutrition (comprising chronic, acute, and vitamin and mineral deficiencies).

Inadequate dietary intake and disease are the immediate causes of undernutrition. Each is described in greater detail in this chapter. These immediate causes relate to Pillar 3 of the Global Action Plan (that is, cost-effective, direct nutrition interventions are scaled up, where applicable).

Underlying these immediate causes are three domains that are a focus of this assessment: (a) food security, (b) health services and health environment, and (c) care for women and children. GAP Pillar 4 emphasizes these domains as they relate to the multisectoral approach required to address key underlying determinants of nutritional problems.

**Figure 3.1    The UNICEF Framework for the Causes of Malnutrition**

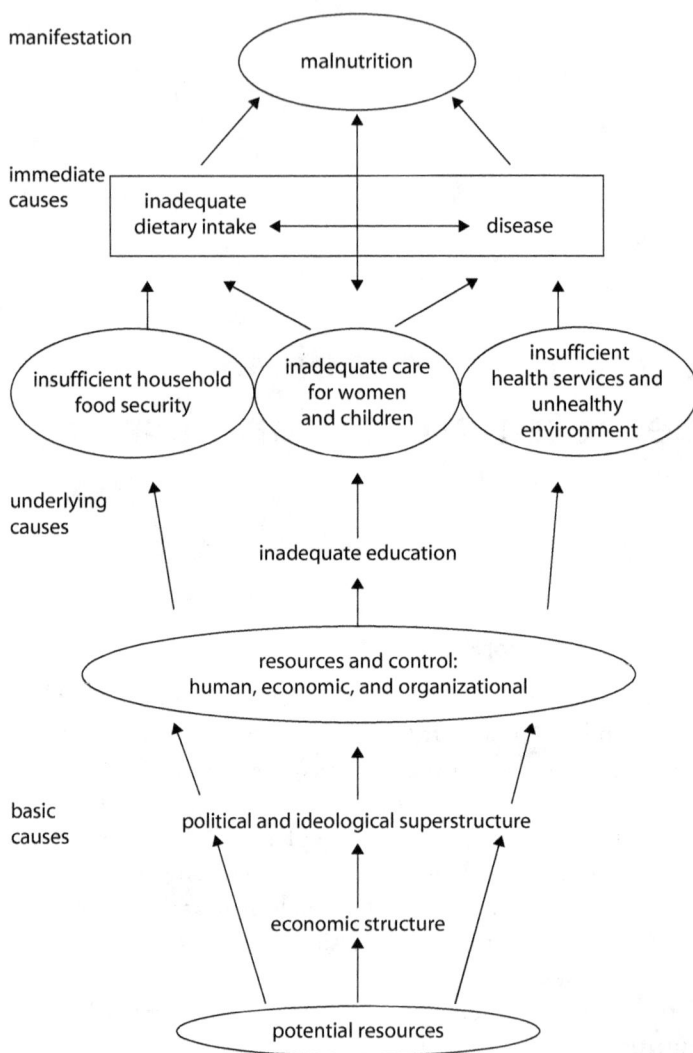

manifestation

malnutrition

immediate causes

inadequate dietary intake ←→ disease

insufficient household food security

inadequate care for women and children

insufficient health services and unhealthy environment

underlying causes

inadequate education

resources and control: human, economic, and organizational

basic causes

political and ideological superstructure

economic structure

potential resources

*Source:* UNICEF 1990.

At the base of the framework are a host of interrelated causes, including resources, economic structure, political and ideological structure, and formal and informal institutions. Although an exhaustive analysis of these causes is beyond the scope of this assessment, they are addressed in GAP Pillar 1 (that is, nutrition is recognized as foundational to national development); Pillar 2 (that is, adequate local capacity is built and supported to design and execute effective nutrition policies and pro-grams); and Pillar 5 (that is, coordinated support for nutrition is provided by development partners).

## Food Security: Inadequate Access and Availability of Food

*Food security* is understood as "when all people, at all times, have physical and economic access to sufficient, safe and nutritious food to meet their dietary needs and food preferences for an active and healthy life" (World Food Summit 1996). National data related to food security come from the National Risk and Vulnerability Assessment (NRVA) for 2003, 2005, and 2007/08 and from the Household Consumption Survey for March 2007. Afghanistan is primarily a rural country whose food security is closely tied with domestic agricultural production. According to the NRVA 2007/08 (CSO 2009a), 69 percent of rural and 55 percent of all households had access to land. Cereal production—particularly wheat—is essential to subsistence because it provides staple food (CSO 2009a). See box 3.1.

According to the NRVA 2007/08, 36 percent of the Afghan population lives below the poverty line. The drastic increase in food prices since 2007 (over 100 percent on some markets); the very harsh winter of 2007/08, which led to 10 percent livestock losses; and drought have con-tributed to deteriorating economic and food security conditions. Growing political insecurity in a number of regions adversely affects food security by reducing households' access to markets and goods. Political insecurity also limits humanitarian agencies' abilities to deliver assistance in most insecure areas. Figures 3.2 and 3.3 illustrate changes in food commodity prices from 2007 to 2009. Wheat prices have recovered from the 2008 food crisis to close to 2007 levels, whereas meat prices have shown a slight increase over that period.

---

**Box 3.1**

### Cereal Deficits in Afghanistan

Even in good production years, Afghanistan experiences a cereal deficit. Although the estimated harvest in 2007 was the highest in the past decade, the cereal deficit was estimated at 220 metric tons.

*Source:* FAAHM 2009.

**Figure 3.2    Local Wheat Prices in Different Regions of Afghanistan, September 2007–September 2009**

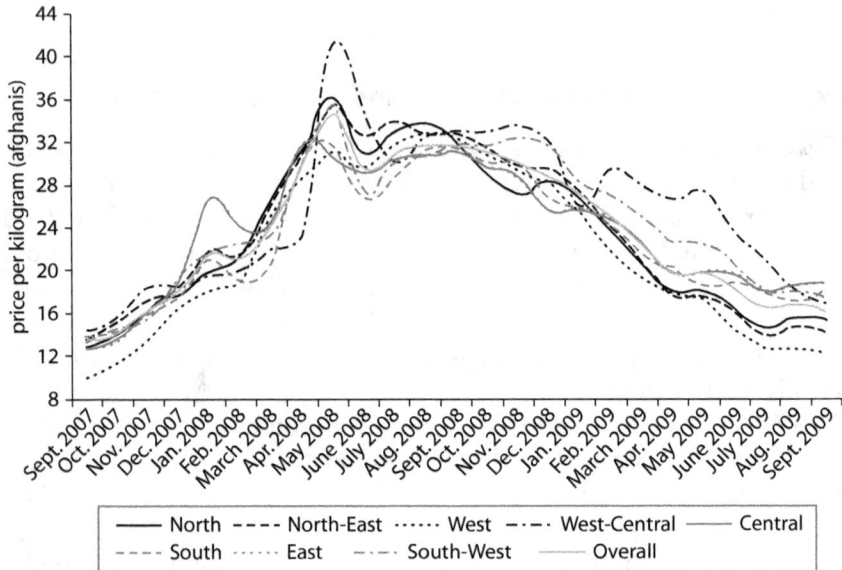

*Source:* Food, Agriculture, and Animal Husbandry Information Management Unit, Ministry of Agriculture, Irrigation, and Livestock, Afghanistan.

Dietary data are available from NRVA surveys, although different methods were used in each successive round, which prevents trend analysis. Consumption patterns were measured through individual interviews with the household's main food preparer. Information is available for household aggregates only. The dietary adequacy data include 2,100-kilocalorie diets as an adjusted estimate of the dietary needs of adults and children. Caloric consumption data show approximately a quarter of households as food insecure across the surveys. Diet diversity data are lacking, particularly national-level studies during a vulnerable season. NRVA studies do show at least a quarter of households as having low diet diversity whether rural only (more vulnerable) or postharvest (optimal time for food diversity). An analysis of NRVA 2003 rural data found that vegetable consumption was low across all socioeconomic strata (Johnecheck and Holland 2005). In the most recent NRVA (2007/08), over a quarter of households (28 percent) had inadequate caloric intake (figure 3.4), but diet diversity was not reported (CSO 2009a).

**Figure 3.3    National Average Price of Beef, Mutton, and Chicken, September 2007–September 2009**

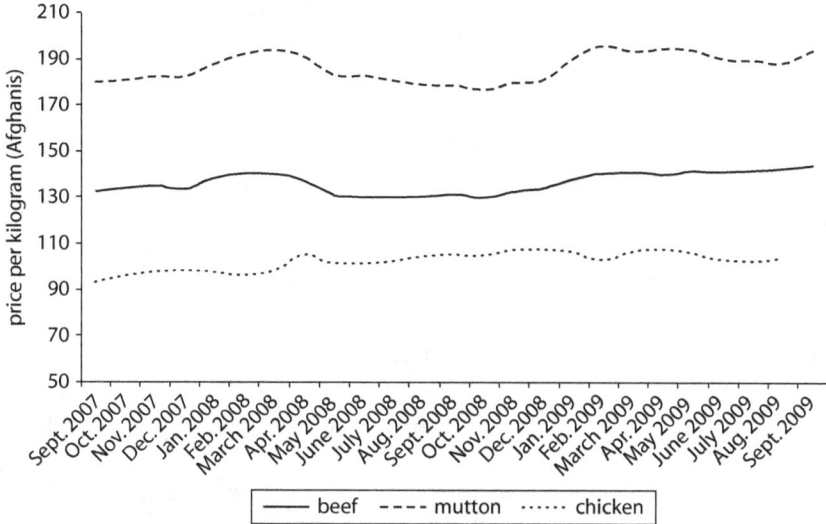

*Source:* Food, Agriculture, and Animal Husbandry Information Management Unit, Ministry of Agriculture, Irrigation and Livestock, Afghanistan.

**Figure 3.4    Household Food Insecurity in Afghanistan, 2003, 2005, and 2007/08**

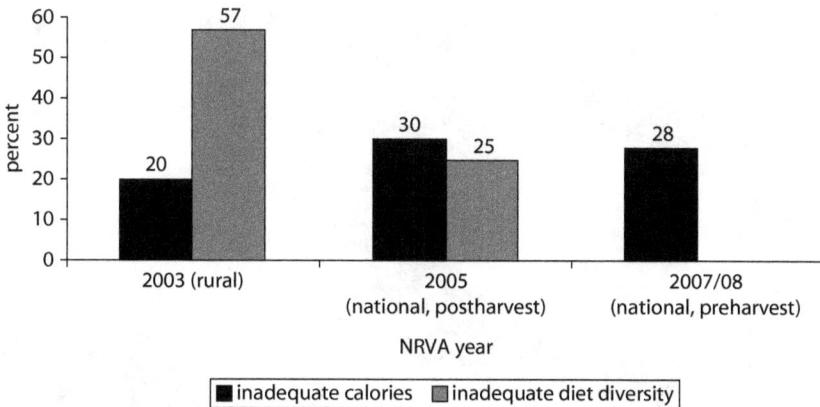

*Source:* NRVA data.
*Note:* Data are not comparable because different methods were used across studies.

Food insecurity occurs seasonally in Afghanistan. Most households are food secure for part of the year but food insecure for other vulnerable months. December through March are reportedly the most challenging months—when food stores are depleted, crops are planted, and little off-farm labor is available for income.

Maps from the NRVA 2007/08 were unavailable. The NRVA 2005 data showed that, along with Nuristan province to the east, the provinces with worst food diversity were located in the central highlands (map 3.1). These areas have poor-quality roads, and access to markets is difficult throughout the year. Provinces in the northern region showed greater diet diversity related to higher and more diversified local production.

The World Food Programme identified highly food insecure regions, particularly in west-central (greater than 85 percent) and north (greater than 60 percent) Afghanistan, as recently as December 2008 (figure 3.5). Other regions report figures closer to the national numbers of around 30 to 40 percent.

For the most vulnerable sectors of the population, a review of Afghan agriculture policy found that the problem is rarely food availability, particularly in markets, but rather inadequate assets with which to purchase food (Christoplos 2004). Drought, crop pests, diseases, and reduced

**Map 3.1    Population Consuming a Diet with Low Food Diversity, by Province, 2005**

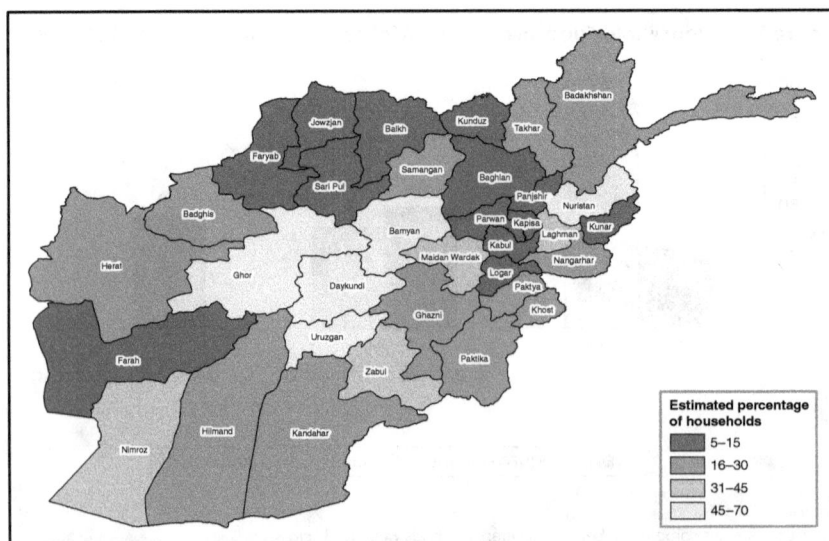

*Source:* NSS 2007.

**Figure 3.5    Percentage of Households with Poor Food Consumption, by Region, August 2007 and December 2008**

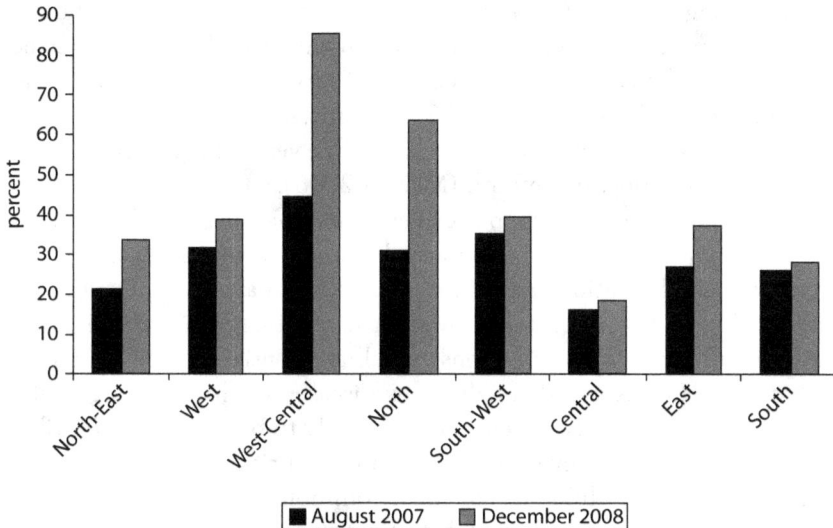

*Source:* World Food Programme Food Security Monitoring System data.

landholdings because of population growth have constrained farmers' cultivation capacity and income generation from agriculture.

Remote areas of Afghanistan may have reduced access to diverse foods. Households with greater access (shorter distance) to markets showed greater diet diversity than those with less market access (Johnecheck and Holland 2005).

Regional food security studies have been conducted by the Food and Agriculture Organization of the United Nations (FAO), Cornell University, the Afghan Ministry of Public Health (MOPH), UNICEF, and the World Food Programme to fill a gap in understanding of local food beliefs and practices. Selected results related to infant and young child feeding (IYCF) are presented in appendix C. Additional data on local food beliefs are available from FAO-Afghanistan, the Ministry of Agriculture, Irrigation, and Livestock's Home Economics Department, and Cornell University.[1]

## Health and Health Services

Undernutrition compromises the immune system's ability to fight infectious disease. Infectious disease, in return, affects nutritional status through its impact on appetite, nutrient loss through decreased dietary absorption (for example, diarrhea); blood loss (for example, helminth infection); or destruction of cells (for example, malaria).

According to the 2004 National Nutrition Survey (MOPH and others 2009), 36 percent of women and 46 percent of children had diarrhea sometime in the two weeks preceding the survey (table 3.1). These data are similar to those of the 2006 Afghanistan Health Survey, which showed that 47 percent of children under five years of age (U5) had diarrhea during the previous month (MOPH 2006).

Data on helminth infection prevalence are unavailable, although given the high frequency of interaction with livestock in rural areas and of poor hygiene and sanitation, helminth and other parasitic infections are expected to be highly prevalent. Malaria control has been enacted in the eastern and other lowland regions, which are considered at high risk for this disease. Levels of other infectious diseases are high among Afghan women and children. Persistent illness is likely to be a primary contributing cause of the high levels of chronic undernutrition and micronutrient deficiencies among children. The most common causes of U5 child mortality in Afghanistan are neonatal deaths (26 percent), acute respiratory infections (25 percent), diarrhea (19 percent), measles (6 percent), and malaria (1 percent) (MOPH 2006).

Trend data illustrate that acute undernutrition appears seasonally concurrent with spikes in diarrhea cases (from poor hygiene, sanitation, and access to potable water) rather than inadequate food (map 3.2). A study conducted in 2003 to 2004 found no association between cases of acute undernutrition and socioeconomic status (Johnecheck and Holland 2005).

**Table 3.1    Prevalence of Morbidity in Children, Women, and Men, 2004**

| Indicator | Children 6–59 months old (%) | Nonpregnant women 15–49 years old (%) | Pregnant women 15–49 years old (%) | Men 18–60 years (%) |
|---|---|---|---|---|
| Diarrhea (3 or more loose or watery stools per day or blood in the stool in previous 2 weeks) | 46.2 | 35.7 | 23.0 | 17.0 |
| Respiratory illness (reported illness with cough, fever, or difficulty breathing in previous 2 weeks) | 40.9 | 23.8 | 40.9 | 30.9 |
| Edema (bilateral pitting) | 2.0 | n.a. | n.a. | n.a. |

Source: MOPH and others 2009.
Note: n.a. = not applicable.

**Map 3.2    Percentages of Households with Access to Safe Drinking Water, by Province, 2007/08**

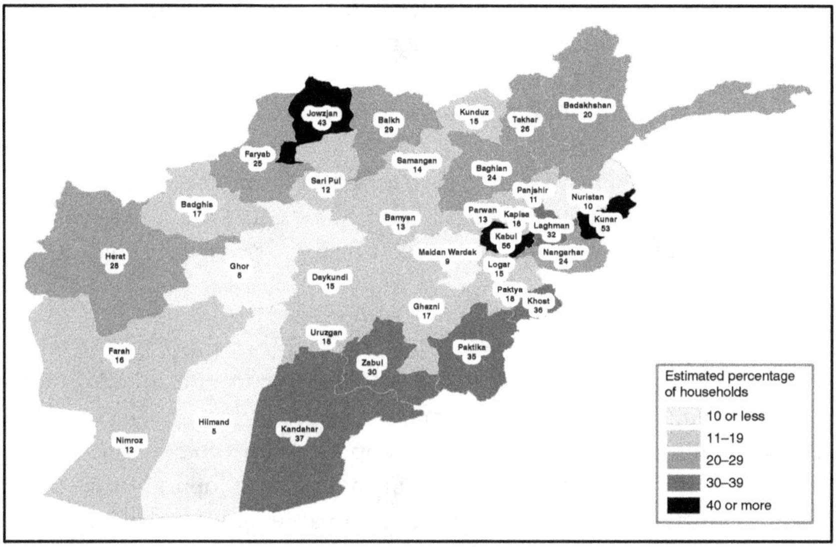

*Source:* CSO 2009a.

Acute undernutrition levels were highest in the 6 to 29 months age group. According to Action Contre la Faim, in winter acute undernutrition often presents with respiratory illnesses.

Although 65 percent of the population now can access primary health care services within one hour by some form of transportation (a dramatic improvement in recent years from 9 percent in 2000), many households still do not have the means to make optimal use of these facilities, and gross differences exist in access by province (CSO 2009a). The government of Afghanistan, with support from the World Bank, the U.S. Agency for International Development (USAID), and the European Commission, extends a Basic Package of Health Services (BPHS) to the population. The BPHS operates through a nationwide network of four types of health facilities: (a) health post, (b) basic health center, (c) comprehensive health center, and (d) district hospital. The health post is staffed by a community health worker (CHW). Each CHW, a resident of the community where he or she serves, generally serves a population of 1,000 to 1,500 individuals. CHWs are hired in pairs (typically one male, one female) to adhere to local customs. See appendixes D and E for a summary of BPHS services.

Distance and cost are reportedly the major barriers to accessing health care. One-way public transportation costs Af 100 (approximately US$2) on average. Private transportation can be four times more expensive. Women and girls often require a male relative for traveling, which doubles travel costs. "Of all girls and women who are ill or injured, 47 percent cite distance and 49 percent cite expenses as a reason for not seeking medical care" (CSO 2009b, 14).

Therapeutic feeding unit monitoring data showed 40 percent of admitted children are younger than six months of age, which suggests that breastfeeding difficulties are a major cause of undernutrition (figure 3.6).

## Health Environment

Poor hygiene, poor sanitation, and limited access to safe drinking water are major contributing causes of infections in Afghanistan. Hygiene conditions within the home or home compound are often poor. Animals reside close to the household. Open latrines may be found in the streets. Map 3.2 illustrates geographic differences in access to safe drinking water by province according to NRVA 2007/08 data.

**Figure 3.6    Comparison of the Number of Admissions to Supplementary Feeding Centers and the Number of Diarrhea Cases Diagnosed in Maternal and Child Health Clinics, August 2001–August 2003**

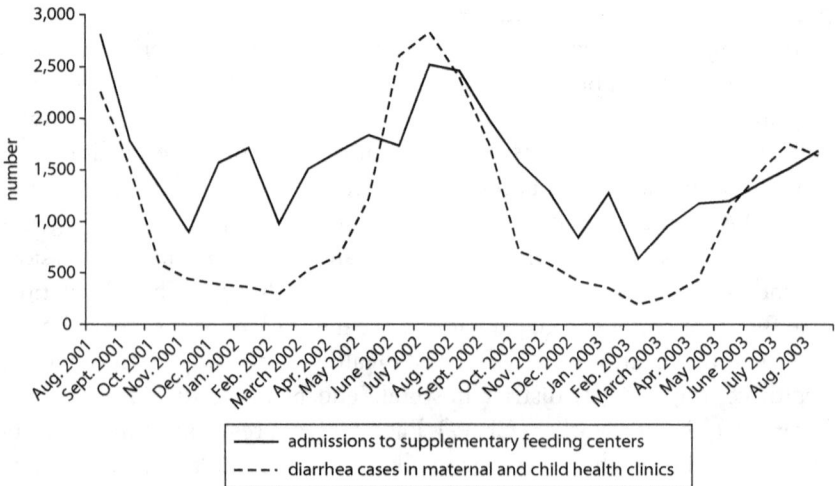

*Source:* Action Contre la Faim data.
*Note:* Supplementary feeding clinics and maternal and child health clinics were operated by Action Contre la Faim.

The NRVA 2007/08 found that only 27 percent of all households had access to safe drinking water, an increase of 5 percent from the NRVA 2005 (CSO 2009a). Despite the greater security problems, the southern and other less secure provinces have greater access to safe drinking water than the more peaceful provinces. This seeming paradox is in part due to the funding stream for water, hygiene, and sanitation activities, which has been biased toward the volatile areas.

NRVA 2007/08 data show only 5 percent of Afghan households having improved sanitation (for example, latrines). No maps are yet available from the recent survey, but earlier NRVA data from 2005 on prevalence of latrines show a geographic pattern similar to that of safe drinking water access, with greater presence in the south and some eastern provinces (map 3.3). The northwestern region also shows higher levels than the central and northeastern regions.

## Care for Women and Children

Poor maternal nutrition locks families into an intergenerational cycle of undernutrition. Stunted or underweight women are at risk of having babies

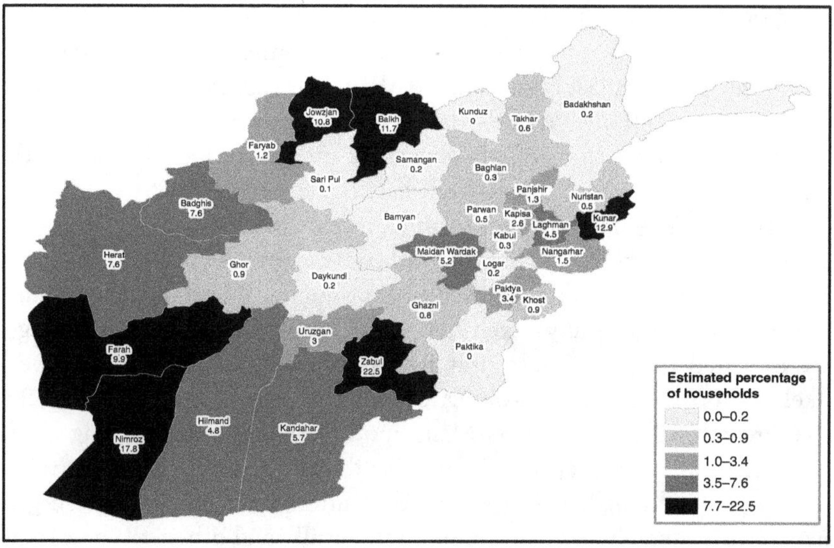

Map 3.3    Percentages of Households with Access to Improved Sanitation, by Province, 2005

with low birth weight. Poor child growth can continue into adulthood, per-petuating the cycle. High rates of underweight and anemia among women—and related vitamin and mineral deficiencies during reproductive years—highlight the necessity of improved care for Afghan women.

According to the NRVA 2007/08, only 36 percent of women access prenatal care, and 15 percent (13 percent rural, 28 percent urban) use contraceptives (CSO 2009a). Prenatal care often does not begin until the third month. This late start leads women to access iron and folate supple-ments only in the second trimester. Iron and folic acid supplementation is critical during the first trimester, when neural tube defects can be pre-vented. The higher incidence of spinal cord defects in Kabul hospitals may be related to this delayed start of supplement use (if supplements are used at all) and to the low coverage of preventive measures such as forti-fication of wheat flour with folic acid.

### IYCF Practices

Inadequate IYCF practices are a major contributing cause of chronic and acute undernutrition in children. In the 2004 National Nutrition Survey, 98 percent of mothers reported breastfeeding their preschool child (6–59 months) at some time (MOPH and others 2009). Over half of chil-dren (60 percent) received mother's milk in the first two hours after birth. More than a third of the mothers (35 percent) of preschool children dis-carded their colostrum prior to initiating breastfeeding. Table 3.2 compares these data with those from other surveys on IYCF since 2002.

Data on exclusive breastfeeding and complementary feeding patterns cover the previous 24 hours only. Although these indicators are World Health Organization standards, data tend to overestimate the proportion of exclusively breastfed infants over a six-month period because of the 24-hour-recall method. Exclusive breastfeeding is believed to be rare in Afghanistan. The data are quite varied, in part because of different sam-pling frames (national compared to convenience samples in selected provinces) and methodologies. Given that qualitative studies have found that few mothers (if any) exclusively breastfeed, the higher percentages are assumed to be accurate only as 24-hour recalls. The other surveys likely included additional probing to bring the figure closer to true exclu-sive breastfeeding prevalence. Many mothers begin breastfeeding a few days after childbirth, reportedly because they do not believe colostrum is healthy for their babies. In the first days after birth, mothers often give newborns water, glucose, juice, nonhuman milk, and other soft and tradi-tional foods (box 3.2). The use of ritual prelacteal foods—such as ghee,

**Table 3.2  Overview of Survey Results on IYCF Practices**

| Source | Coverage | Initiation | Breastfeeding | | | Complementary feeding | |
|---|---|---|---|---|---|---|---|
| | | | Exclusive breastfeeding among children 0–6 months (%) | Percentage breastfed at 1 year | Percentage breastfed at 2 years | Age of introduction (months) | Percentage fed at that age |
| Afghanistan Health Survey 2006 | National | 37% in first hour | 70 | — | — | 6–9 | 28 |
| National Nutrition Survey 2004 | National | 60% within 2 hours; 92.8% within 12 hours; 35% discarded colostrum | — | — | — | — | — |
| Multiple Indicator Cluster Survey 2003 | National | 92.7% in first day | — | 91 | 54 | 6–9 | 28 |
| 2003 survey by UNICEF | Herat | 59.2% in first hour; 82.2% use colostrum | 19.4 | 93 | 34 | 6–9 | 71 |
| 2002 survey by UNICEF and the U.S. Centers for Disease Control and Prevention | Badghis | — | 95 | 96 | 52 | 6 | 21 |
| 2003 survey by UNICEF and MOPH | Parwan | — | 12.5 | 64 | 63 | 6–9 | 40 |
| 2002 survey by Save the Children USA | Jowzjan | About 50% fed colostrum | 0 | — | — | "Most mothers had introduced foods or liquids at 4 months." | |

Source: Authors' compilation based on unpublished survey data.
Note: — = not available.

---

**Box 3.2**

## Predominant Breastfeeding

*Predominant breastfeeding* better characterizes current population practices during the early months of life. In predominant breastfeeding, breast milk is the main source of nourishment for the infant; however, certain liquids (water, tea, juices, ritual drinks) are also given.

*Source:* WHO 2008.

---

herbs, or even dirt—is common, and tea or watery soup may be given earlier than six months, jeopardizing the healthy development of infants.

Bottle feeding and pacifier use are common in urban and, increasingly, rural areas. Poor knowledge of bottle hygiene, flies, and a scarcity of clean drinking water significantly increase the potential risk of infection through bottle feeding. Pacifiers are often clipped to the child's clothing but may become dirty through contact with others' hands and clothing.

Most women breastfeed for one year, and about half breastfeed for two years. Cultural beliefs and mental health both play a critical role in breastfeeding practices in Afghanistan. Many women believe that breast milk is *haram* (impure, dirty) when they become pregnant or ill. This belief leads some of them to wean their child at an early age. Mothers also often claim to have insufficient breast milk. Problems with lactation are associated with depression or other mental health issues. MOPH officials cite levels as high as 66 percent of Afghans having depression.[2] Many caregivers—and even health staff—have come to believe that breast milk insufficiency is normal. This belief also results in part from low levels of awareness about appropriate breastfeeding techniques (for example, proper positioning), particularly those that can stimulate the production of breast milk. The experience of insufficient breast milk can result from early cessation of breastfeeding because of the beliefs described (though reinitiation can trigger lactation again) and low awareness of problem-solving techniques.

Only a third of infants tend to be introduced to solid or semi-solid (complementary foods) at the proper age of six months. Surveys specific to introduction at six months are lacking. Formative research has been gathered to inform interventions by Cornell University, MOPH, UNICEF, and Save the Children USA and experience through trials of improved practices (FAO and Ministry of Agriculture, Irrigation, and Livestock).

This research shows that caregivers often introduce complementary foods too early, too late or both. Young children often are fed from the family plate, rather than receiving specific dishes suited to their needs. They rarely receive a separate ration that they can eat at their own pace. Complementary foods are often inadequate, consisting essentially of watery soups that lack energy-dense protein and micronutrient-rich foods. Caregivers do not feed children frequently enough, and quantities often fail to meet children's nutritional needs. Appendix C provides information from an FAO study on cultural beliefs about foods helpful or harmful for young children.

In May 2009, stakeholders concerned with IYCF gathered for a workshop organized by the MOPH (with support from FAO, Save the Children USA and U.K., UNICEF, the USAID Basic Support for Institutionalizing Child Survival (BASICS) III Project, USAID, the World Food Programme, and the World Health Organization) on the preparation of a national strategic plan for infant and young child feeding. Participants from these and other stakeholder groups in the MOPH, other ministries, and non-government organizations identified the nine chief constraints to adequate IYCF listed in box 3.3.

### Women's Mental Health

Three decades of civil conflict have taken a toll on families, leading to reduced social support networks, early death, reduced assets, debt, and

---

**Box 3.3**

### Key Constraints to Optimal IYCF Practices in Afghanistan

- Low knowledge and skills related to optimal IYCF practices
- Traditional beliefs and food taboos
- Lack of peer support
- Limited resources such as time, food, and the like
- Mothers' poor nutrition and health status
- Early marriage and pregnancy
- Mothers' workload
- Low birth spacing
- Influence of commercial products (in particular breast milk substitutes and commercial complementary feeding porridges)

*Source:* National IYCF strategy workshop, Kabul, May 2009.

increased vulnerability to natural and human-made shocks. Mental health support is rare in Afghanistan but has been included in the revised BPHS. Upholding one's family's honor is central to Afghan culture. Thus, admitting mental health problems (for example, symptoms of depression, anxiety, and posttraumatic stress disorder) and seeking care can be culturally challenging. Social support networks for women are limited. Women are generally prevented from attending religious worship because the mosque is largely the domain of men; rather, women are encouraged to worship within the home compound. Women are permitted to visit relatives and neighbors within the community. Women's groups also play a critical function in providing a social support resource for Afghan women. Nevertheless, whether the problem is societal (for example, violent conflict or threats) or domestic (for example, abuse), most women suffer quietly. Mental health challenges adversely affect mothers' capacity to care for their children (for example, by providing breastfeeding, responsive complementary feeding, or play to support child motor and cognitive development).

## Nutrition Awareness

Basic nutrition has not been promoted systematically nationwide. As a result, no simple illustration, such as a food group guide for obtaining a balanced diet, is available to share with the public. The Public Nutrition Department has focused on specific topics rather than a more general nutrition message. Awareness about vitamins in the Afghan population was reported in the 2004 National Nutrition Survey (MOPH and others 2009). In a general sense, 33 percent of men and 16.5 percent of women stated that they knew about vitamins. No significant differences in vitamin awareness were found among men or women by age. For both genders, those who were literate and educated were more likely to have heard of vitamins than those who were illiterate ($p < 0.05$) *and those who were uneducated* ($p < 0.05$). Most men and women believed that vitamins "give strength." Other responses included that vitamins make people healthier, prevent and treat illness, and increase intelligence. The NRVA 2007/08 reports that only 17 percent of the population over age 25 has had any formal education, and only 26 percent are literate. Half (52 percent) of eligible children attend primary school. Low levels of female literacy (12 percent) are well recognized as contributing to undernutrition.

Many policy makers feel that traditional cultural beliefs about food and household food allocation patterns play an important role in Afghan diets (Levitt, Pelletier, and Pell 2009). Qualitative research in northern Afghanistan on household food allocation revealed no systematic differences in terms of quality or quantity of food allocated to men compared to women or children in Tajik communities. According to local women, each household member received some of each type of food available (for example, meat, vegetables, and fruit); husbands sometimes received a greater portion, but women and children both received a sizable allocation (Levitt, Stoltzfus, and others 2009). This issue requires further exploration in other regions and ethnic groups.

A hot-cold food belief system is pervasive throughout Afghanistan and affects feeding practices of all family members. Research in northern Afghanistan suggests that the hot-cold food belief systems may relate to the heat produced through metabolism of the food. For example, foods that have higher calorie density (for example, sugars and fats) were often characterized as "hot" or "warm" in comparison with those that were more water based (for example, many vegetables) or less calorific. Additional research is warranted to further understand this important determinant of local food beliefs and practices. These food beliefs have important implications for nutrition promotion programs.

Multiple family members influence how women feed themselves and their children. In an FAO study in three provinces (Bamyan, Badakhshan, and Herat) and one study in Balkh province,[3] women reported various sources of advice about nutrition. These sources included relatives (elders, mothers, mothers-in-law), "experienced people," "educated or literate people," literacy teachers, trainings, religious instructors, health workers (doctors, midwife or *daya*, other), and radio and television. Other family members, particularly mothers-in-law, influenced mothers' decisions about how to feed themselves and their children; this finding indicates the importance of targeting messages to families as a whole. A mother's consumption of healthy foods often is restricted by food taboos (particularly during pregnancy and lactation), poor knowledge of women's nutritional requirements, limited resources, limited decision-making power, and mothers' tendency to focus on other family members' needs before their own.

## Summary

Maternal and child undernutrition in Afghanistan is clearly caused by a combination of determinants. At least a third of Afghan households experience food insecurity, and half have inadequate diet diversity. Frequent illness and challenges in accessing health care lead to nutrient losses, especially in women and infants. Low use of prenatal care and contraceptives put women at increased health risk. IYCF practices are inadequate. Nutrition knowledge is scarce.

However, not all underlying factors will necessarily be present for a given population in a specific geographic area. Thus, the specific determinants of undernutrition in a given area (for example, in a district or province) will need to be assessed (for example, through the standardized nutrition survey recommended in chapter 2). Once the causes of undernutrition in that geographic area are identified, a selection of the interventions that are proposed in subsequent chapters of this report can be tailored to address the main causes.

A useful way to carry out this analysis within a geographic area is to make the following determinations in a stepwise fashion:

1. Is food is available in markets (production, trade)?
2. Do households have access to the food (affordability)?
3. Is the available food of adequate quality (diversity, micronutrients, safety)?
4. Is the food properly used by women and children (feeding practices for women and young children)?
5. Is the food that is eaten well absorbed (infections, helminths)?

An analysis using these questions follows a hierarchical path. For example, in a geographic area where food security is a problem, this issue needs to be addressed before or at the same time as other factors, such as feeding practices and infections.

This chapter has shown that some of the determinants, such as food availability, vary significantly across provinces in Afghanistan and in different seasons. Although this report outlines the broad causes of undernutrition in Afghanistan, such analysis of determinants will need to be carried out at the provincial and district levels to design a comprehensive yet tailored response that addresses the most important determinants. The menu of responses is discussed in chapter 5. Whereas some responses will likely need to be national (for example, increasing access to water and sanitation or increasing access to micronutrients), others (for example, improving food availability and access) will be confined to certain areas.

## Notes

1. Unpublished data are available from research in Balkh province during 2006 to 2007 from Emily J. Levitt (EJL5@cornell.edu).

2. Personal communication, Dr. F. Kakar, Ministry of Public Health, General Directorate of Primary Health Care and Preventive Health, Kabul, July 22, 2009.

3. Unpublished research by FAO-Afghanistan; research in Balkh was conducted by Emily J. Levitt of Cornell University (EJL5@cornell.edu).

## References

Christoplos, Ian. 2004. "Out of Step? Agricultural Policy and Afghan Livelihoods." Afghan Research and Evaluation Unit, Kabul.

CSO (Central Statistics Office). 2009a. *National Risk and Vulnerability Assessment 2007/08: A Profile of Afghanistan*. Kabul: Ministry of Rural Rehabilitation and Development.

———. 2009b. "Summary of the National Risk and Vulnerability Assessment 2007/8: A Profile of Afghanistan." Ministry of Rural Rehabilitation and Development, Kabul.

FAAHM (Food, Agriculture, and Animal Husbandry Information Management and Policy Unit). 2009. "Agriculture Prospects Report." FAAHM, Ministry of Agriculture, Irrigation, and Livestock, Kabul.

Johnecheck, Wendy, and Diane Holland. 2005. "Nutritional Risk in Afghanistan: Evidence from the NSS Pilot Study (2003–2004) and the NRVA 2003." Tufts University, Medford, MA.

Levitt, Emily J., David L. Pelletier, and Alice N. Pell. 2009. "Revisiting the UNICEF Malnutrition Framework to Foster Agriculture and Health Sector Collaboration to Reduce Malnutrition: A Comparison of Stakeholder Priorities for Action." *Food Policy* 34 (2): 156–65.

Levitt, Emily J., Rebecca J. Stoltzfus, David L. Pelletier, and Alice N. Pell. 2009. "A Community Food System Analysis as Formative Research for a Comprehensive Anemia Control Program in Northern Afghanistan." *Food Security* 1 (2): 177–95.

MOPH (Ministry of Public Health). 2006. *Afghanistan Health Survey 2006: Estimates of Priority Health Indicators for Rural Afghanistan*. Kabul: MOPH.

MOPH (Ministry of Public Health), UNICEF (United Nations Children's Fund), CDC (Centers for Disease Control and Prevention), National Institute for Research on Food and Nutrition–Italy, and Tufts University. 2009. *2004 Afghanistan National Nutrition Survey*. Atlanta: CDC.

NSS (National Surveillance System). 2007. *The National Risk and Vulnerability Assessment 2005: Afghanistan*. Kabul: Ministry of Rural Rehabilitation and Development and Central Statistics Office.

UNICEF (United Nations Children's Fund). 1990. "Strategy for Improved Nutrition of Children and Women in Developing Countries: A UNICEF Policy Review." New York: UNICEF.

WHO (World Health Organization). 2008. "Indicators for Assessing Infant and Young Child Feeding Practices: Part 1—Definitions." WHO, Geneva.

World Food Summit. 1996. "Rome Declaration on World Food Security and World Food Summit Plan of Action." Documents signed at the World Food Summit held by the Food and Agriculture Organization of the United Nations, Rome, November 13–17. http://www.fao.org/wfs/index_en.htm.

# CHAPTER 4

# Political Economy and Capacity to Address Undernutrition

Given that the causes of malnutrition originate in multiple sectors, good nutrition cannot be achieved by one sector alone. However, to expect multisectoral action (that is, joint implementation by various sectors in the same geography) in Afghanistan, where the institutional capacity for service delivery is still weak, would be unrealistic. A more realistic approach is to plan multisectorally but act sectorally (World Bank 2007). For example, there should be a national nutrition plan that envisages a clear and specific role for key sectors that translates into sector-specific plans. Each sector would then implement its plan and coordinate with other sectors on a periodic basis (for example, during an annual results conference).

This chapter examines the political economy, institutional structures, and implementation arrangements currently in place in Afghanistan to address undernutrition in relevant sectors. The capacity of these structures and arrangements to implement effective, scaled-up nutrition interventions is also assessed. Two pillars of the Global Action Plan for Nutrition directly relate to this analysis (box 4.1; see chapter 1 for background on the Global Action Plan).

The first pillar is the degree to which nutrition has achieved sufficient salience in the policy arena to be positioned as a foundation to national development. The following question is posed: Does nutrition

**Box 4.1**

## Pillars of the Global Action Plan Pertinent to National Infrastructure for Nutrition

*Pillar 1:* Nutrition is recognized as foundational to national development [political economy, institutional arrangements].

*Pillar 2:* Adequate local capacity is built and supported to design and execute effective nutrition policies and programs [implementation arrangements and capacity].

*Source:* "Scaling Up Nutrition (SUN): A Framework for Action."

have high-level support in the central government? The second pillar involves the following question: Does existing central-level support (of whatever magnitude) translate to a strong policy and programming infrastructure and capacity for provincial and lower-level implementation?

## Pillar 1: Nutrition Is Recognized as Foundational to National Development

The Afghanistan National Development Strategy (ANDS) is the main strategic planning document of the government of Afghanistan. It is the country's poverty reduction strategy, organized with the goal of helping Afghanistan achieve all of the Millennium Development Goals. In the ANDS, the government's priorities are outlined through 2013. The extensive consultation process that led to the ANDS included involvement of many development stakeholders: line ministries, provincial authorities, community leaders, development partners, United Nations (UN) agencies, and nongovernment organizations (NGOs). Nutrition and food security are most directly addressed in the ANDS Health and Nutrition Sector Strategy (HNSS) and the Agriculture and Rural Development Sector Strategy (ARDSS), with attention to a lesser degree in the Social Protection Sector Strategy (SPSS) and Education Sector Strategy (ESS).

The HNSS largely focuses on the priorities of the Ministry of Public Health (MOPH) and the mechanisms for providing health services through contracting arrangements to NGOs. Although the Ministry of Agriculture, Irrigation, and Livestock (MAIL) is a cosignatory of the HNSS, food security issues are addressed primarily through the ARDSS. Food safety and quality control overlap, although these mechanisms have yet to be clearly defined. Both ministries are expected to liaise with the Afghanistan National Standards Authority of the Ministry of Commerce (MOC), which has recently emerged to oversee safety and quality control of food and other commercial commodities. As a result, neither the HNSS nor the ARDSS can serve as Afghanistan's overarching, multisectoral national nutrition strategy document. The MOPH and the MAIL each have their own respective policies related to public nutrition and food security.

Although Afghanistan has no separate national, cross-cutting nutrition strategy, precedent exists for initiating something of this nature, given that six cross-cutting strategies already exist within the ANDS framework (capacity building, gender equity, counternarcotics, regional cooperation, anticorruption, and environment), each with multiple ministries as cosignatories (see appendix F). The cross-cutting strategies serve to harmonize other ANDS sectoral strategies and frame the links to the broader national development objectives. Establishing a cross-cutting nutrition strategy would also facilitate the formation of a high-level committee (for example, a consultative group) to plan and coordinate nutrition policies and programs for Afghanistan. In the HNSS (MOPH and MAIL 2008, 21) the current Consultative Group on Health and Nutrition (CGHN) is described as follows:

> **Consultative Group on Health and Nutrition:** The central platform to maximize the coordination and integration of all related activities of the [Health and Nutrition Sector] to promote a common approach to assessing sector problems and provide guidance, direction, and overall advisory leadership.

The strength of the system of ANDS and consultative groups is that they provide the needed high-level planning and coordination mechanism for development in the country. The current limitations of the HNSS and CGHN are that they are highly health sector oriented but include limited participation from the other ministries, apart from agriculture, working to support nutrition. The HNSS and CGHN could be strengthened to provide the required multisectoral support for nutrition at the national level, but such action would require bringing other ministries (besides the MAIL) under the HNSS as cosignatories to allow for required oversight authority Such cosignatories might include the following ministries: the Ministry of Rural Rehabilitation and Development (MRRD); Ministry of Women's Affairs; Ministry of Commerce; Ministry of Mines and Industry; Ministry of Justice; Ministry of Labor, Social Affairs, Martyrs, and Disabled (MOLSAMD); Ministry of Education; Ministry of Higher Education; and Ministry of Religious Affairs.

## The Health and Nutrition Sector Strategy

Despite the prominence of the word *nutrition* in the HNSS, the document focuses largely on primary health care concerns. One of the 18 strategies is to "Reduce prevalence of malnutrition and increase access to micronutrients," and Public Nutrition is listed as one of the five core Health Care Service Provision Programs in the country (MOPH and MAIL 2008, 24). However, the MOPH's Public Nutrition Department (PND) is not given a position in the MOPH structure parallel to the four other programs that are designated as directorates (Reproductive Health and Child Health, Hospital Care, Primary Health Care, and Disease Control). Nutrition appears as a subcomponent of the Primary Health Care directorate, categorized as a part of the Basic Package of Health Services (BPHS). Active lobbying was required to ensure nutrition objectives were included explicitly in the HNSS rather than solely as subcomponents of other broader programs. The challenge facing the PND, which mainstreams many of its activities through other MOPH programs (for example, vitamin A through the National Immunization Days, and iron and folic acid supplementation through prenatal care), is to maintain visibility outside these other programs.

Development partners in Afghanistan also have not accorded nutrition the relative priority it should have, given its effect on national development. Some development partners (for example, Canada and the United States) have funded nutrition programs, but these investments represent a small fraction of their overall contributions. As this report outlines later, the BPHS is one of the platforms through which health sector nutrition services can be delivered, but to date the BPHS has not prioritized nutrition interventions. The revised BPHS package contains most well-proven health sector nutrition interventions, but they are not prioritized during implementation (for example, the coverage of iron and folic acid supplementation through the BPHS is not measured).

Thus, to date, political commitment, positioning within the MOPH structure, and resource allocation by the government of Afghanistan and development partners for public nutrition remain inadequate, compared to its importance for socioeconomic development and political stability (appendix G). As such, despite the stated HNSS goal and MOPH mission statement (box 4.2), nutrition is not currently recognized as foundational to national development by high-level HNSS stakeholders.

Despite these limitations, compared to many countries, Afghanistan has an impressive and innovative staffing and coordination infrastructure designed to support nutrition. The nutrition policy process was catalyzed

**Box 4.2**

## HNSS and MOPH Mission Statements

The goal of the HNSS is

[T]o work effectively with communities and development partners to improve the health *and nutritional status* of the people of Afghanistan, with a greater focus on women and children and under-served areas of the country." (emphasis added)

The mission of the Ministry of Public Health is

[T]o improve the health *and nutritional status* of the people of Afghanistan in an equitable and sustainable manner through quality Health Care Service Provision and the promotion of a healthy environment and living conditions along with living healthy life styles." (emphasis added)

*Source:* MOPH and MAIL 2008, 5.

by the publication of a U.S. Agency for International Development (USAID) food security assessment that described Afghanistan's situation as a "cash famine" (Lautze and others 2002). The report highlighted how financial, food, and asset securities all decreased by more than 70 percent from 1999 to 2002, reducing Afghans' capacity to cope with natural and human-made shocks. On the basis of this assessment and a desk review of available studies, the research team recommended a public nutrition (multisectoral) approach to address the broad economic and sociopolitical causes of food insecurity and undernutrition in the country (Assefa and others 2001; Dufour and Borrel 2007). The government responded to this report with a request for greater nutrition programming. The public nutrition approach involves addressing each of the domains illustrated in the United Nations Children's Fund (UNICEF) framework for the causes of undernutrition (see chapter 3).

Although in 2002 capacity was weaker in other sectors, the MOPH supported setting up a PND that would both carry out direct nutrition interventions and coordinate actions to address certain multisectoral determinants of undernutrition (see box 4.3). The PND was established in the MOPH in late 2002. UNICEF invited Tufts University to assist in building nutrition capacity in the MOPH. Tufts worked with a three-year capacity-building grant from the American Red Cross to support two full-time staff members and consultants, who worked in the MOPH alongside the PND staff. The MOPH provided four national nutrition officers. Over

**Box 4.3**

## The Public Nutrition Approach

As described in the first Public Nutrition Policy and Strategy (MOPH and Tufts University 2003), the public nutrition approach is designed to help populations

- Address underlying causes, involving sectors of food security, health, and care for mothers and children
- Reflect the social, cultural, and political context
- Build on community capacities and skills
- Apply lessons learned from other countries and guidelines that are considered to be best practice

These best practice guidelines are intended to be used to inform program and policy design for Afghanistan and to be adapted to this context. UNICEF's conceptual framework for the causes of malnutrition, which highlights the interrelationships between food, health, and care, served as the basis for this policy. This policy "represents a paradigm shift from clinic-based treatment of malnutrition to the broader food security, social and care environment, and the public health aspects addressing the underlying causes of malnutrition" (MOPH and Tufts University 2003, 2).

*Source:* MOPH and Tufts University 2003.

the period from 2003 to 2005, a cadre of 34 provincial nutrition officers (PNOs) were hired and trained to oversee policy and program implementation (see appendix I for PNO job description). Although the PND does not have authority over other ministries, the staff coordinated multisectoral activities through a host of thematic working groups.

Current national policies in nutrition and food security all have their basis in the Public Nutrition Policy and Strategy (PNPS) of 2003–06, the first such policy developed by the PND. The PNPS adopted the holistic public nutrition approach, emphasizing direct nutrition interventions as well as additional domains of key determinants of undernutrition: food security, health services, health environment, and care for women and children. This policy contrasted to earlier programming, which focused on specific health sector interventions (for example, iron and folic acid supplementation and breastfeeding promotion). Within this framework, the nutrition community compiled existing nutrition data from regional surveys; interviewed key stakeholders in nutrition-relevant institutions (for example, UNICEF provincial offices, and various NGOs); and determined seven priority thematic issues. A working group was created for each priority issue:

- Surveys and surveillance (food security and nutrition)
- Micronutrient deficiencies
- Maternal and child nutrition
- Community-based food security and food aid
- Management and treatment of severe acute undernutrition
- Prevention and management of acute malnutrition and chronic malnutrition
- Capacity building in public nutrition

The working groups invited involvement from officials in other government ministries (for example, the MAIL, MRRD, Ministry of Women's Affairs, Ministry of Education, and MOC); national and international NGOs; and UN agencies. Each working group provided specific technical recommendations for policies, strategies, and activities related to its priority area. The PNPS process and document laid a foundation for interministerial partnerships, an approach that continued in successive policy processes. Subsequent to the publication of the PNPS and its translation into both local languages (Dari and Pashto), the working groups transitioned to become task forces to assist the PND (which was ultimately responsible) with oversight of the PNPS. PNOs were to mobilize similar task forces at the provincial level. Countries rarely have a structure like the PND, which mobilizes its staff to think and work in a multisectoral fashion despite being situated in one sector.

In 2009, with support from the USAID Basic Support for Institutionalizing Child Survival (BASICS) III Project, the PND updated its policy for 2009 to 2013 through a multisectoral consultative process (similar to that used in 2003). The new document is titled the *Public Nutrition Strategy (PN Strategy) 2009–2013*, with the term *policy* removed at the request of the MOPH Policy and Planning Department because the entire MOPH is to have one overarching policy to which the departmental strategies contribute. Also during 2009, and before the completion of the Public Nutrition Strategy, two related nutrition strategy documents emerged: the Strategy on Prevention and Control of Vitamin and Mineral Deficiencies in Afghanistan, developed with technical assistance from the Micronutrient Initiative (see box 5.3 in chapter 5), and the National Infant and Young Child Feeding (IYCF) Strategy, developed with support from BASICS (see box 5.4 in chapter 5). The vision, goal, and overall objective of the Public Nutrition Strategy are noted in box 4.4.

Box 4.5 includes guiding principles of the new Public Nutrition Strategy. Priorities in the strategy for 2009 to 2013, updated from the 2002 list, include the seven priority challenges shown in box 4.6. Appendix K presents a table of the corresponding priorities with their respective strategies and implementing partners. The top priority relates to increasing knowledge and skills about nutrition in the population. Other priorities modified from the earlier policy include a stronger focus on community-level programs and enhanced data collection capabilities. Continuing priorities include attention to IYCF, micronutrients, treatment and prevention of moderate and severe acute malnutrition, and capacity building of public nutrition personnel. The revised Public Nutrition Strategy aims to address these seven challenges by building on current achievements and interventions.

### The Agriculture and Rural Development Sector Strategy

Under the ANDS framework, the agriculture sector contributes to nutrition through both the HNSS and the ARDSS. The two ministries active in this sector are the MAIL and the MRRD. The ARDSS discusses nutrition briefly in the context of human food security (and nutrition of livestock). It mentions the percentage of the population not meeting basic dietary needs, using National Risk and Vulnerability Assessment (NRVA)

---

**Box 4.4**

**Guiding Features of Afghanistan's Public Nutrition Strategy, 2009–13**

*Vision:* All Afghans are protected from all forms of malnutrition, by benefiting from optimal food intake, feeding and caring practices, and health, nutrition, and hygiene services.

*Goal:* To protect and promote healthy nutrition for all Afghans, to prevent chronic malnutrition and associated micronutrient deficiency disorders, and to reduce mortality from acute malnutrition, in particular among mothers and children.

*Overall objective:* To increase access to and use of quality nutrition services provided at the community level and through health facilities.

*Source:* MOPH 2009.

**Box 4.5**

# Guiding Policy Principles of the Public Nutrition Strategy, 2009–13

These guiding policy principles are inspired by the public nutrition approach, which was adopted in the first Public Nutrition Policy and Strategy 2003–2006, and by the guiding principles in the general MOPH Policy and Strategy 2005:

- *Addressing the multiple underlying causes of undernutrition.* The causes of undernutrition are manifold and context specific. Reducing undernutrition requires treating symptoms while also addressing underlying causes (such as food insecurity, poor feeding and caring practices, and poor health and hygiene) by implementing preventive interventions.
- *Understanding political, economic, social, and cultural factors.* The categories of underlying causes are determined by economic, agricultural, and trade policies. Additionally, cultural and social norms influence people's ability to access food as well as their food consumption patterns. The MOPH will advocate for policies that protect the population's nutritional status and design interventions that are adapted to cultural and social norms.
- *Encouraging multisectoral collaboration.* Undernutrition cannot be effectively addressed through health interventions alone. Professionals from a broad range of sectors—such as health, agriculture, economy, education, and rural development—should contribute to the design and implementation of programs in public nutrition.
- *Using community-based interventions and civil society participation.* Participation of local communities and civil society stakeholders, including the private sector, is essential for effectiveness and sustainability. The Public Nutrition Strategy prioritizes interventions that should be implemented at the community level, targeted at vulnerable population groups and households.
- *Ensuring sustainability and use of local resources.* Nutrition interventions should as much as possible be based on the promotion of locally available resources, to reduce the risk of dependency on foreign products. Interventions should be designed to be sustainable and replicable by local communities.
- *Promoting integration in all levels of the health system.* Nutrition interventions that are implemented through the health system need to be integrated at all levels of health care, from community level with community health workers and community support groups to provincial hospitals. All health personnel have a responsibility for promoting good nutrition practices.

*(continued)*

**Box 4.5** *(continued)*

• *Using evidence-based interventions and action-oriented strategies.* Assessments to describe the extent and severity of the problem of undernutrition, including a description of the risks and causes, must be conducted to inform the design or revision of interventions. A process of learning is required that is evidence based and involves wide dissemination of lessons learned and demonstration of translating policies into practice.

*Source:* MOPH 2009.

**Box 4.6**

## Priority Nutrition Challenges for Afghanistan, 2009–13

1. Inadequate knowledge and skills for achieving good health nutrition
2. Inadequate IYCF and limited community outreach of current IYCF counseling and support
3. Low micronutrient intake and poor dietary diversity, associated with low coverage and limited quality of current micronutrient interventions
4. Presence of severe acute undernutrition and limited access to quality treatment
5. Low availability of reliable nutrition data
6. Inadequate response to moderate acute malnutrition
7. Limited capacity in public nutrition among health practitioners and professionals from other nutrition-related sectors (agriculture, education, social affairs, and so on)

*Source:* MOPH 2009.

data; the high prevalence of chronic undernutrition among children (more than 50 percent); and the high level of iron deficiency among women and children (more than 70 percent), citing National Nutrition Survey data. In section 3 of its policy framework, the ARDSS states:

**Assurance of food security**: The Government is responsible to establish a viable and sustainable food security system, promoting dietary diversification for better *nutrition*, and mitigating the effects of crop failure and/or animal diseases. Short term food security (food aid) should be provided in extreme circumstances and if required it can be provided through food/cash for work programs. (emphasis added) (Islamic Republic of Afghanistan 2008, 20)

Although the statement for nutrition is an important step politically, direct support for nutrition or food security programs remains weak. Many view food security as a given outcome of improved agricultural systems, and thus the latter gain most attention.

In 2004, six development partners agreed to collaborate on agriculture sector development: the Asian Development Bank, the U.K. Department for International Development, the European Commission, USAID, the U.S. Department of Agriculture, and the World Bank. The agreement required that the MAIL elaborate a detailed agriculture sector development strategy—a "master plan" to guide investment. The master plan included a full chapter dedicated to food security, prepared with technical support from the Food and Agriculture Organization of the United Nations (FAO). After a change of ministers in 2008, the master plan was reworked into a National Agriculture Development Framework (NADF). The programs relevant to nutrition or food security in the NADF are listed in box 4.7. A food security chapter was not incorporated into the NADF.

The nutrition components of the NADF fall primarily under the Agriculture Production and Productivity program. The nutrition-related programs in existence are largely those set up during the master plan process (2005–07). In 2006, FAO led a Food Security Working Team in developing the food security components of the master plan. Reconvening the Community-Based Food Security Task Force that had been set up by the MOPH's PND, FAO used the public nutrition approach, taking advantage of existing malnutrition data from the PND policy for the food security planning process. The food security community also adopted the UNICEF malnutrition framework to highlight the links between food

---

**Box 4.7**

## The Four Programs of the NADF

- Agriculture Production and Productivity (staple crops, fruits, vegetables, livestock products and industrial crops)
- Natural Resource Management
- Economic Regeneration (includes quality control and food safety)
- Change Management, Public Sector Development, and Program Support Framework

*Source:* MAIL 2009, 4.

security, diet, and nutritional status. FAO's preexisting food security projects, conducted in partnership with the MAIL, were deemed appropriate administrative structures for more permanent government nutrition and food security activities.

One FAO staff person was assigned to explore how to mainstream food security in the NADF programs. Another FAO project focused on capacity building within the MAIL (Household Food Security, Nutrition and Livelihoods 2005–2010) and also worked to support mainstreaming of nutrition and food security through MAIL programs as well as gender mainstreaming. Through this German-funded project, FAO has employed a full-time expatriate nutritionist within the MAIL. The project works directly with the MAIL's Home Economics Department (HED), originally a unit of the extension department and still within the extension system. The HED receives technical and operational support from FAO and is staffed primarily by women. The HED's focus is to fill the gap in basic nutritional knowledge and skills among the general population and to support household food security in rural areas. Of note, this goal is also the top priority in the new Public Nutrition Strategy. This overlap is no coincidence, because the MOPH's PND and the MAIL's HED work closely on nutrition planning and promotion (for example, joint material development, joint trainings of trainers). Both departments contribute technically, with support from international partners, and each department has different channels for dissemination. The MOPH has wider access to rural communities through its facilities, but the MAIL could play an important role at the village level (see box 5.6 in chapter 5 for an alternative approach in the health sector for mobilizing communities).

Similar to the PNO structure, the FAO and the HED jointly recommended hiring female extension workers, or home economics officers, at the provincial level. The creation of two positions in each province was approved in late 2006, and the recruitment process was launched in 2007. These officers are assigned to collaborate with the PNOs to support harmonization of provincial activities, including training.

The FAO-HED project focuses its activities mainly in four provinces where resources are available for programming: Bamyan, Badakhshan, Herat, and Kabul. As of the end of 2008, through training-of-trainers strategies and collaboration with local NGOs, nutrition promotion activities reached approximately 30,000 households. The project has worked through NGO literacy teachers, community health workers, and agriculture extension agents. Chapter 5 provides additional information about these specific programs.

Continued advocacy efforts and technical assistance are required to ensure that food security and nutrition concerns are effectively mainstreamed in agricultural development efforts. Advocates will need to be vigilant to see that interventions for household food security (not just national food security) are supported. This effort specifically involves ensuring that (a) projects are targeted at the most vulnerable—and often underserved—areas and households; (b) agricultural projects support diet diversification and income generation, not just cereal production; and (c) households gain the knowledge and skills required to recognize the crops and animal products necessary for a balanced diet and the knowledge and skills needed to prepare, preserve, and use adequate food.

A joint program has been created between the health and agriculture ministries, as well as their partner UN agencies, to accomplish these three objectives. It is the only large-scale multisectoral nutrition program of its kind in Afghanistan. The program has received partial funding from the Spanish Millennium Development Goals Trust Fund (see chapter 5).

The MRRD is the MAIL's main partner in addressing food insecurity and poverty reduction. Table 4.1 presents the MRRD's many large-scale programs. The MRRD is not currently involved in core nutrition discussions; however, representatives attend broader policy discussions and participate in working groups, particularly those related to food security surveillance. The MRRD oversees the NRVA. The MRRD also plays a central role in improving access to safe drinking water, sanitation, and hygiene education. Given the importance of surveillance, safe water, sanitation, and hygiene to nutrition and the current very low rates of coverage, the MRRD should be a key partner in a multisectoral approach to nutrition in Afghanistan. MRRD programs provide an available platform for numerous other interventions (for example, nutrition promotion), but their strongest contribution will likely be in improving access to safe drinking water, sanitation, and hygiene education.

### The Social Protection Sector Strategy
The SPSS identifies nutrition concerns such as food insecurity and malnutrition during natural disasters and in the broader context of addressing the needs of chronically vulnerable groups. Reducing childhood undernutrition (underweight) is noted as one of the benchmarks of the Afghanistan Compact, and links are made in the SPSS to increasing support to poor households with young children. A reduction in child underweight is included as an outcome indicator of SPSS programs.

**Table 4.1    Nutrition-Relevant Programs in the MRRD**

| Program | Activities | Potential areas of collaboration on nutrition |
|---|---|---|
| National Surveillance System | In collaboration with the Central Statistics Office, the National Surveillance System conducts the NRVA. | Through the NRVA surveys, the National Surveillance System could collect data every round on underlying causes (household food security, maternal and child care, health service access, health environment) and every other round on individual nutrition indicators (subsample for women, children, men). |
| National Solidarity Program | The program has established approximately 22,000 community development councils throughout the country, with support from facilitating partners (NGOs). These councils implement local microdevelopment projects (mainly infrastructure) and serve as the main conduit and coordination body for development interventions at village level. | Men's and women's councils could be a platform for nutrition promotion activities. The National Solidarity Program is one of the main vehicles for improving water, hygiene, and sanitation. |
| Rural Water, Sanitation and Irrigation Program | The program provides a safe water source, demonstration latrines, hygiene and health education (including in schools), and small-scale irrigation projects. | The program directly supports communities with a package of services, including safe drinking water, latrines, and hygiene education. |
| National Area-Based Development Program | The program provides support to district-level governance (institutionalization of district development assemblies), rural infrastructure services, and small-scale economic regeneration activities. | These MRRD programs provide economic support for vulnerable households. Nutrition promotion (for example, complementary feeding) may have little effect in highly food insecure households without providing some support for food acquisition (for example, livelihood support or cash transfer). |
| Afghan Rural Enterprise Development Program (in process) | The program is designed to support micro- and small enterprises for rural income generation. | Nutrition projects in food insecure areas should partner with economic support activities. |
| Microfinance Investment Support Facility | This facility is now a separate government agency supporting microfinance institutions. | |

*Source:* Authors' compilation.

Poor nutrition is also identified as a concern among other vulnerable groups. The MOLSAMD works with several groups: (a) martyrs' families, (b) those with war-related disabilities, (c) orphans and children enrolled in kindergartens, (d) victims of natural disasters, (e) pensioners, and (f) the unemployed. A decrease in the number of individuals who suffer from hunger is included as an outcome indicator of SPSS programs, measured through the NRVA. The SPSS defines *food poverty* as measured by a household's inability to acquire a basic food basket providing 2,100 kilocalories per person. This degree of food poverty is experienced by 28 percent of Afghans, according to the NRVA 2007/08 report (CSO 2009). Nutrition-relevant programs sponsored through the MOLSAMD are described in chapter 5. No interaction with the PND was discerned at present.

### *The Education Sector Strategy*
The ESS highlights the importance of nutrition for preschool and school-age children (MOE 2008). The government of Afghanistan currently provides kindergarten and nursery (crèche) facilities to allow female employees to return to work after childbirth. Facilities provided are similar to those in the private sector. The ESS recommends strengthening support for nutrition of preschool children through early childhood development programs in these facilities, because only day-care service is provided. The Ministry of Education also receives food assistance from the World Food Programme for school feeding programs (1 million tons wheat, in the form of high-protein biscuits). This program, for which India is a major development partner, operates in 31 provinces (all except Badghis, Kabul, and Panjshir). A Healthy Schools Initiative also exists, whose focal activities pertain to water, hygiene, sanitation, deworming, landmine safety, and improved educational quality. No nutrition education is yet included. The Ministry of Higher Education oversees Kabul Medical University, which includes some nutrition topics in its curriculum. USAID has funded a broad, capacity-building Higher Education Project through the Academy for Educational Development, subcontracted to the University of Massachusetts Amherst Medical School. The design is to assist with revising the undergraduate medical curriculum, to add a nutrition course, and to develop a master's of public health program including at least one nutrition course. FAO staff members have given nutrition lectures to students in the Faculty of Agriculture at Kabul University. These lectures have been very popular, reportedly drawing standing-room-only attendance.

### Other Ministries Contributing to Nutrition

Other ministries that support nutrition include the Ministry of Energy and Water, the Ministry of Women's Affairs, the Ministry of Religious Affairs, the Ministry of Commerce, the Ministry of Mines and Industry, and the Ministry of Justice. Relevant activities of these ministries are shown in table 4.2.

### Gaps and Opportunities Identified Pertaining to Pillar 1

A number of challenges and opportunities have been identified pertaining to Pillar 1:

- The strategic importance of improved population nutrition is not well appreciated in any sector, nor are sufficient resources allocated to have a significant influence. This situation is particularly problematic in the health, agriculture, and rural development sectors, as evidenced by the constant advocacy required by nutrition and food security stakeholders during the ANDS planning process. Although nutrition is now prominently included in the HNSS and ARDSS policies, political and

**Table 4.2    Other Ministries with Activities Supportive of Nutrition**

| Ministry | Activities |
|---|---|
| Ministry of Women's Affairs | Women's community groups (women's *shuras*[a]) are a platform for literacy, health, and nutrition education and income-generation projects (with support from NGOs). |
| Ministry of Energy and Water | Large-scale irrigation projects and energy supply (for example, cooking fuel) are the purview of this ministry. |
| Ministry of Religious Affairs | This ministry plays a key role in public-awareness campaigns and community mobilization through mullahs, mosques, and respected Muslim leaders. |
| Ministry of Commerce and Ministry of Mines and Industry | These ministries partner with the MOPH for the enforcement of the Code of Marketing of Breast Milk Substitutes (MOC) and Universal Salt Iodization campaign (both ministries). They are key partners for increasing private sector contributions in nutrition. In addition, MOC supports the Afghanistan National Standards Authority for food safety and quality control (domestic and imported fortified foods). |
| Ministry of Justice | The ministry is involved with any legislation (for example, Code of Marketing of Breast Milk Substitutes, maternity legislation) and regulations regarding food and nutrition. |

*Source:* Interviews with representatives from nutrition partners, who cited participation of these ministries in nutrition activities.

a. *Shura* is the traditional term used to designate a community council or an assembly.

operational support for programs remains weak. No national costed action plan exists for nutrition (with targets), nor do sufficiently ambitious action plans exist within relevant ministries. Without such action plans, policies will not attract the necessary resources to transform the visions outlined in documents into actions that will improve nutritional status.

- Given the low coverage rates of access to safe water, to improved sanitation facilities, and to hygiene education, insufficient priority has been given to accelerating the scale-up of MRRD's Water, Sanitation, and Irrigation Program. Whether partnerships with the private sector (for example, social marketing of water treatment kits) have sufficiently been explored is not clear.

- Although the MOLSAMD may recognize the strategic importance of nutrition, it is in a weaker position technically and operationally to implement large-scale programs. Building strategic (informal or formal) alliances with the MOLSAMD, the Ministry of Education, the MRRD, and the MOC, among others, may be important for the MOPH's PND and the MAIL's HED to increase their standing within their own respective ministries. Currently, these alliances are formal in the HNSS between the health and agriculture sectors but informal in other instances (such as coalitions for advocacy around issues of joint concern).

- The example of the six cross-cutting ANDS issues provides a model and precedent for developing a cross-cutting policy and a corresponding high-level coordination committee (for example, consultative group) for nutrition. Such an approach would provide a mechanism within the existing national policy structure to have a national nutrition policy that is situated above separate ministry policies but that includes and harmonizes content of those respective policy documents. If this model were pursued, it would require firm, multiyear commitments from development partners to avoid the risk that the HNSS might drop the "N" for "Nutrition" from its title.

- Research in 2006 and 2007 among policy makers revealed that support for nutrition was not weak because of lack of interest but rather because of lack of familiarity with maternal and child nutrition issues, lack of understanding of the effect of nutrition on health and development, and unfamiliarity with nutrition-related interventions. Support from development partners for other interventions also biased policy makers' focus to other issues (Levitt and others 2009).

- Opportunities exist for the MOPH and the MAIL to strengthen nutrition for early childhood development in partnership with the education and social protection sectors.

## Pillar 2: Adequate Local Capacity Is Built and Supported to Design and Execute Effective Nutrition Policies and Programs

Despite support provided by some development partners to improve the government of Afghanistan's capacity to design and execute nutrition policies and programs, significant capacity gaps remain. Most support has focused on building the capacity of the MOPH's PND and the MAIL. Detailed analysis of the current capacity and gaps within the MOPH and MAIL can be found in appendix I. The methodology used in this report to carry out the capacity assessment of the two ministries is described by Potter and Brough (2004). This capacity assessment uses a four-tier hierarchy of capacity-building needs:

1. Structures, systems, and roles
2. Staff and facilities
3. Skill
4. Tools

Tier 1 (structures, systems, and roles) forms the base of the capacity structure, with each successive tier (tiers 2, 3, 4) building on the previous one.

As explained earlier in this report, the MOPH has received support from partners such as Tufts University, UNICEF, the World Health Organization (WHO), the World Food Programme (WFP), FAO, and the Micronutrient Initiative to enhance its capacity to design and execute effective nutrition policies and programs. The early support led to the creation of the PND. However, the PND is weakly positioned within the MOPH and has no real authority over partners to enforce agreements pertaining to nutrition. System capacity constraints also exist relating to information and financial flows as well as capacity to contract services. Staff members attend in-service and short-course trainings that equip them to implement existing programs but have taken no formal degree courses in nutrition. Strong technical support is often provided for programs from development partners: all activities generally require support from outside organizations (for example, FAO, the Micronutrient Initiative, UNICEF, WFP, or WHO). Technical support is routinely requested for policy revision and other programmatic strategic planning activities. Moreover, the PND has difficulty retaining provincial and some national staff members because of low salaries and inadequate operational support to complete functions of the job description. Security and severe weather conditions during parts of the year make in-country travel and communication problematic. The PND receives support from partners that fund projects for some monitoring activities. The lack of departmental transportation (owning a vehicle or renting a car and driver) hampers both provincial and national personnel in monitoring activities. A clear indication of the PND's weak capacity is the relatively low priority accorded to the delivery of nutrition interventions in the BPHS, as noted earlier.

The MAIL suffers from similar capacity constraints but is currently receiving more direct support than is the PND. The main department focusing on direct nutrition interventions is the MAIL's HED. The HED differs from the MOPH's PND in that it has an on-site UN partner organization, FAO, providing daily capacity-building support. The PND began with this model, from 2003 to 2005, when Tufts University consultants were placed in the MOPH to work directly with PND officers. The HED and FAO counterparts participate or take the lead in task forces and ANDS consultative group meetings. These meetings can make corporate decisions, but they have limited ability to hold partners accountable to commitments related to nutrition or food security through existing structures. Collaborations succeed depending on the strengths of social networks and relationships. FAO support allows adequate communications and transportation, which facilitate flows of information and resources. Managerial decisions are made in a timely manner because bureaucratic delay between the national and provincial staffs is limited. Because the HED benefits from direct FAO support, private sector contractors may be hired if FAO approves. Staff members are learning in-service and through study tours the skills required for their work. FAO also provides training sessions as well as day-to-day in-house capacity-building support for HED national officers. No HED officers have formal degree training in nutrition. Staff members have a reasonable mastery of their project-related knowledge from multiple years' experience. However, technical support is still requested for strategic planning and policy, research, and program management.

Perhaps the greatest capacity gap is the weak program infrastructure to carry out community-based nutrition. Although the BPHS front-line workers—the community health workers—could have been positioned to carry out community nutrition activities, this role currently encompasses too many job responsibilities (three-page terms of reference); as a result, not much of their time is spent on community nutrition activities. The MAIL offers training-of-trainer activities that should eventually lead to increased knowledge and improved behaviors at the community level, but it is not clear that the full program results chain (that is, from training-of-trainers to interactions with communities) has been fully planned yet. Other countries in the region (for example, Nepal and Pakistan) have systems of community workers or volunteers who spend a significant amount of time addressing nutrition issues at the community level with a focus on behavior change. Such models have yielded positive effects and could be considered to enhance the capacity for nutrition programming at community level in Afghanistan.

Continuing to build capacity within the MOPH and MAIL will be important, but addressing capacity gaps in the MRRD will also be critical, particularly to enable the acceleration of scale-up of safe drinking water, improved sanitation, and better hygiene. Addressing the overall nutrition system capacity—for example, the national capacity to plan multisectorally for nutrition, implement sectorally, and then review results and lessons learned again multisectorally—will be important. Elements of that system are currently in place (for example, for policy formulation), but some capacity gaps exist (program planning and execution, results monitoring, and review). The capacity of the government to harness the resources and abilities of the private sector in Afghanistan to improve nutrition will also need to be enhanced (for example, marketing of nutrition products and nutrition-enhancing behaviors and regulation of fortification of foods).

## References

Assefa, Fitsum, Mohammed Zahir Jabarkhil, Peter Salama, and Paul Spiegel. 2001. "Malnutrition and Mortality in Kohistan District, Afghanistan, April 2001." *Journal of the American Medical Association* 286 (21): 2723–28.

CSO (Central Statistics Office). 2009. *National Risk and Vulnerability Assessment 2007/08: A Profile of Afghanistan.* Kabul: Ministry of Rural Rehabilitation and Development.

Dufour, Charlotte, and Annalies Borrel. 2007. "Towards a Public Nutrition Response in Afghanistan: Evolutions in Nutritional Assessment and Response." In

*Reconstructing Agriculture in Afghanistan,* ed. Adam Pain and Jacky Sutton, 93–118. Warwickshire, U.K.: Practical Action.

Islamic Republic of Afghanistan. 2008. *The Agriculture and Rural Development Sector Strategy.* Kabul: Islamic Republic of Afghanistan.

Lautze, Sue, Elizabeth Stites, Neamat Nojumi, and Fazalkarim Najimi. 2002. "*Qaht-e-Pool* 'A Cash Famine': Food Insecurity in Afghanistan 1999–2002." Feinstein International Famine Center, Tufts University, Medford, MA.

Levitt, Emily J., Rebecca J. Stoltzfus, David L. Pelletier, and Alice N. Pell. 2009. "A Community Food System Analysis as Formative Research for a Comprehensive Anemia Control Program in Northern Afghanistan." *Food Security* 1 (2): 177–95.

MAIL (Ministry of Agriculture, Irrigation, and Livestock). 2009. "Umbrella Document for the National Agriculture Development Framework." MAIL, Kabul.

MOE (Ministry of Education). 2008. "Education Sector Strategy for the Afghanistan National Development Strategy." MOE, Kabul.

MOPH (Ministry of Public Health). 2009. *National Public Nutrition Strategy, 2009–2013.* Kabul: MOPH.

MOPH (Ministry of Public Health) and MAIL (Ministry of Agriculture, Irrigation, and Livestock). 2008. *Health and Nutrition Sector Strategy 1387–1391 (2007/08–2012/13).* Kabul: Government of Afghanistan. http://www.moph.gov.af/en/downloads/Strategy_2007_2008_2012_2013 .pdf.

MOPH (Ministry of Public Health) and Tufts University. 2003. *Public Nutrition Policy and Strategy, 2003–2006.* Kabul: Ministry of Public Health.

Potter, Christopher, and Richard Brough. 2004. "Systemic Capacity Building: A Hierarchy of Needs." *Health Policy and Planning* 19 (5): 336–54.

World Bank. 2007. *From Agriculture to Nutrition: Pathways, Synergies, and Outcomes.* Washington, DC: World Bank.

# CHAPTER 5

# Current Programs, Gaps, and Opportunities

Nutrition is inherently a multisectoral matter, and therefore programs to address undernutrition often involve more than one sector. This chapter covers three pillars described by the Global Action Plan (GAP) for Nutrition (box 5.1). Pillars 3 and 4 address the need for interventions that focus on direct and underlying causes of undernutrition, respectively. Pillar 3 highlights investment in direct nutrition interventions (for example, supplementation, fortification, and nutrition promotion). Many aspects of maternal and child care are included in the direct interventions under Pillar 3 (see box 5.2). Pillar 4 takes a multisectoral approach to tackling undernutrition at the country level and includes activities that address food security, health systems strengthening, hygiene, and sanitation. Pillar 5 emphasizes coordination among development partners to support nutrition.

## Pillar 3: Cost-Effective, Direct Nutrition Interventions are Scaled Up, Where Applicable

There is a critical window of opportunity during prepregnancy up to the first two years of a child's life for averting risk of maternal and child death, and if mother and child survive, for avoiding lifelong harm from

---

**Box 5.1**

## Pillars of the Global Action Plan for Nutrition Relevant to Program Implementation

*Pillar 3:* Cost-effective, direct nutrition interventions are scaled up, where applicable.

*Pillar 4:* Determinants of undernutrition are addressed through multisectoral approaches.

*Pillar 5:* Coordinated support for nutrition is provided by development partners (including funding for advocacy, communications, and research)

*Source:* "Scaling Up Nutrition (SUN): A Framework for Action."

---

**Box 5.2**

## Direct Nutrition Interventions Recommended under Pillar 3

### Prepregnancy and Maternal Nutrition

- Adequate maternal nutrition and prevention of low birth weight: iron and folic acid supplements, vitamin A supplements, multiple micronutrient supplements, protein or calorie supplements (including fortified food), iodized salt, and iron-fortified foods
- Prevention and management of infections: deworming, malaria control, and hygiene promotion (for example, hand washing)

### Infant and Young Child Nutrition

- Adequate infant nutrition: breastfeeding and complementary feeding practices
- Micronutrient investments: vitamin A, iron, zinc, and multiple micronutrient powders
- Management and prevention of severe acute undernutrition
- Prevention and management of infections: deworming and hygiene promotion

*Source:* "Scaling Up Nutrition (SUN): A Framework for Action."

---

inadequate nutrition (figure 5.1). The GAP framework encouraged countries to strive to reduce nutritional problems to the levels in industrial countries and to eliminate vitamin and mineral deficiencies as a public health problem altogether. In humanitarian emergencies, the GAP recommended ensuring delivery of adequate responses, as well as appropriate treatment for severe acute undernutrition. Highlights of the Afghanistan national micronutrient strategy are in box 5.3.

**Figure 5.1    Trends in Prenatal Care Use in Afghanistan, 2003–08**

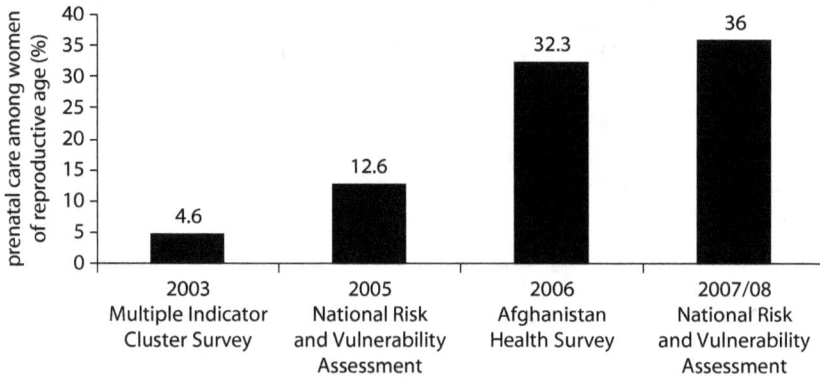

*Sources:* CSO 2009; MOPH 2006; NSS 2007; UNICEF 2003.

**Box 5.3**

# Highlights of the Afghan Strategy on Prevention and Control of Vitamin and Mineral Deficiencies

Based on successful experiences in other countries, evidence from published literature, and the current public nutrition situation and capacity in Afghanistan, recommended strategies follow three broad themes:

- Strengthen micronutrient deficiency prevention (and treatment) programs through the Basic Package of Health Services.
- Expand and strengthen public, private, and civic sector partnerships.
- Develop public and private sector human capacity and expertise.

By the end of 2013, the strategy's objectives are as follows:

- Strengthen national human capacity in nutrition science and food industry to adequately prevent and control vitamin and mineral deficiencies in Afghanistan.
- Sustain 90 percent or greater coverage of high-dose vitamin A capsule distribution among children 6 to 59 months old.
- Enable 90 percent or more of households to regularly access and consume iodized salt.

*(continued)*

**Box 5.3** *(continued)*

- Increase the coverage through the Basic Package of Health Services to 50 percent for iron and folic acid supplementation for pregnant and lactating women and iron supplementation of children under 24 months old.
- Fortify all flour locally produced or imported with vitamins and minerals according to World Health Organization recommendations (iron, folic acid, zinc, vitamin A, and vitamin $B_{12}$).
- Enable 30 percent of households to use commercially or home-fortified complementary foods to feed their children.
- Increase the use of zinc supplementation as a component of diarrhea treatment among 80 percent or more of affected preschool children.

*Source:* MOPH 2009.
**Note:** Importation of oil and ghee fortified with vitamin A (and possibly vitamin D) is also being explored by the Ministry of Public Health in partnership with the Micronutrient Initiative. If feasible, the strategy sets a goal of 90 percent or more households regularly accessing vitamin A–fortified cooking oil and ghee.

The direct nutrition interventions listed in box 5.2 include proven investments that have been widely tested and implemented in many countries. Most have demonstrated potential for high coverage in varied settings. A key challenge for countries is to build sufficient capacity to implement at scale, taking into consideration context-specific implementation challenges, and to maintain high-quality services. These priorities line up well with the priorities of the Public Nutrition Department (PND) of the Ministry of Public Health (MOPH) and the Home Economics Department (HED) of the Ministry of Agriculture, Irrigation, and Livestock (MAIL).

### *Prepregnancy and Maternal Nutrition*
The importance of reaching women before pregnancy with iron and folic acid (IFA) to avert anemia and birth defects is stated in the PND's 2009 strategy:

> Iron and folic acid supplementation should also be considered for adolescent girls and women of reproductive age given the importance of iron and folic acid in the very early stages of pregnancy. (MOPH 2009, 34)

Supplementation with IFA is a core component of prenatal care services through the MOPH's Basic Package of Health Services (BPHS). However, no official programs were identified to intervene prior to pregnancy. Over 90 percent of BPHS facilities reportedly have the capacity to administer proper prenatal care. IFA is supposed to be available free of cost at all levels of the system—health post (home of the community health worker, or CHW); basic health center; comprehensive health center; and district hospital—but coverage of receipt or compliance by women does not exist, so assessing the effective scale of the program is impossible. CHWs also are responsible for referring pregnant women to the nearest health facility for additional care. Facility-level care includes guidance on breast-feeding, birth spacing, safe pregnancies, immunization, health messages, and screening for complicated pregnancies.

The National Risk and Vulnerability Assessment (NRVA) 2007/08 reported that 36 percent of women use prenatal care services. Urban women (71 percent) are more likely to do so than rural women (30 percent), and the percentage is even lower among the nomadic *Kuchi* population (17 percent). Nationally, women who had a primary education were twice as likely to use prenatal care services (67 percent) as those without primary education (33 percent). These figures compare favorably with the 2006 Afghanistan Health Survey (MOPH 2006) data, which showed prenatal care use by 32.3 percent of women with pregnancies in the previous two years. These figures demonstrate a significant increase from 4.6 percent reported in the 2003 Multiple Indicator Cluster Survey (UNICEF 2003; see figure 5.1 for prenatal care trends). In the Afghanistan Health Survey 2006, prenatal care use was associated with having any level of schooling, having higher wealth, and living less than a two-hour walk from a health facility. Despite this encouraging trend, an almost eightfold increase in four years, prenatal care use is still quite low, and data on specific nutrition interventions within the prenatal care package are unavailable.

A focus group with a staff from six BPHS nongovernmental organizations (NGOs) revealed the following programmatic constraints to IFA supplementation:

- Use of prenatal care services is low.
- Most women come for prenatal care services only after the third month (into the second trimester), when IFA still protects against anemia but folate has little effect on preventing birth defects.
- Women (among others in society) are generally unfamiliar with the benefits of IFA.
- Some BPHS staff members prescribe and give IFA without clearly explaining its benefits and side effects.
- Some confusion exists about correct dosage of IFA, and varying dosages were identified in BPHS pharmacies.

Vitamin A supplements are provided through the immunization campaigns for postpartum women and through BPHS facilities. Coverage is consistently below 25 percent.

Maternal protein and calorie supplementation (including fortified food) is currently included in the PND strategy. To address the high levels of maternal underweight, the nutrition community is promoting healthy diets, improvements in household food security, and control of infectious diseases, but little evidence exists to show how much of this information is reaching women or their influencers.

Multiple micronutrient supplements are recommended, where possible, for women of reproductive age. These supplements may be provided through public-private sector partnerships, health facilities, or other mechanisms. No program currently exists for multiple micronutrient supplementation of women (which would replace the IFA supplementation program) in Afghanistan, but within the MOPH, there is interest in considering this intervention.

Deworming during pregnancy reduces iron losses and risk of anemia. Deworming tablets should be available through the BPHS system at all levels (health post to district hospital), but no data are available on current coverage. A survey of 60 households in Balkh province found only one household reporting use of deworming medications for children under five years of age (U5). No mothers had used the medication themselves, despite a wide recognition of the problem of worms (*kerm*) in the community (Levitt, Stoltzfus, and others 2009). Deworming interventions, funded by the United Nations Children's Fund (UNICEF), focus on school-age children (for example, the Healthy Schools Initiative), although anemia and parasite risk remain high in other age groups (U5 children, women of reproductive age, and men) because of poor food hygiene, among other causes.

Use of insecticide-treated bed nets during pregnancy to prevent malaria can reduce risk of low birth weight and anemia. An effective malaria control program is supported through the MOPH for affected areas.

Gaps and opportunities related to improving prepregnancy and maternal nutrition include the following:

• No national programs exist to reach women before pregnancy with IFA, although the PND policy recommends intervention during that time.
• Currently, the level of understanding is low among health service providers, women, and the general public regarding the use (dosage) and benefits of IFA supplements for women of reproductive age.

- No data are available on coverage of or compliance with IFA supplementation. Compliance is likely low, given low use of services. Community-based strategies are probably required to increase compliance once women have accessed prenatal care.
- Use of prenatal care services is low but increasing (36 percent). More than 90 percent of BPHS facilities can provide proper prenatal care, according to the MOPH. Incentives may be needed to encourage women to come for services.

### Infant and Young Child Nutrition

Support for infant and young child feeding (IYCF) programs has been high within the United Nations—including in UNICEF, the World Health Organization (WHO), the Food and Agriculture Organization of the United Nations (FAO), and the World Food Programme (WFP)—as well as within the World Bank and the MOPH's PND. However, only recently has greater attention been paid to infant and young child nutrition in Afghanistan. In 2008, the U.S. Agency for International Development (USAID) through Basic Support for Institutionalizing Child Survival (BASICS) increased its commitment and resources for infant and young child nutrition. From March 29 to 31, 2009, BASICS supported a National Consensus Building Workshop on IYCF. More than 60 participants agreed on policy and programmatic priorities to improve infant and young child nutrition in Afghanistan. Contributors included the MOPH, MAIL, Ministry of Women's Affairs, Ministry of Rural Rehabilitation and Development (MRRD), and Ministry of Commerce, along with colleagues from national and international NGOs, FAO, UNICEF, and the WHO. The workshop was organized with the MOPH and led to the development of the National Infant and Young Child Feeding Policy and Strategy 2009–13, which has been incorporated in the revised Public Nutrition Strategy for 2009–13. Highlights of the IYCF strategy are provided in box 5.4. Current IYCF initiatives supported by the government and its partners are listed in table 5.1. National coverage of these interventions is still minimal (box 5.5).

*Breastfeeding.* The revised BPHS includes many interventions to support IYCF. Prenatal care includes breastfeeding promotion and is a good vehicle even if use is low (36 percent). The Integrated Management of Childhood Illness (IMCI) program includes guidance to mothers on proper breastfeeding and complementary feeding practices. Hospital staff members are also trained in breastfeeding counseling. A training cascade

**Box 5.4**

## Highlights of the National Strategic Plan for IYCF

Based on the recommendations by WHO for optimal infant and young child feeding, Afghanistan's National Strategic Plan for scaling up IYCF activities includes the following:

- IYCF activities—in particular, breastfeeding and complementary feeding counseling—should be clearly integrated at all levels of health services, from the community level (working with CHWs) to provincial and regional hospitals.
- Support groups for mothers should be established, building on existing networks, such as women's community groups, literacy circles, health support groups, and producer organizations. Through these support groups, mothers will receive breastfeeding and complementary feeding counseling and be linked to education and food security interventions that can assist families in accessing more diverse and nutritious foods.
- A harmonized education campaign should be implemented to spread information about adequate feeding practices using a broad range of networks, including religious leaders, teachers, health workers, agriculture extension workers, and community mobilizers.

Adequate policies, guidelines, and funding must support these interventions to ensure that the necessary personnel and training are in place to implement work at the community level. Representatives from various ministries have agreed to work together at the central, provincial, and community levels to garner necessary support and resources to make these plans a reality.

*Sources:* Data from MOPH and USAID BASICS.

has been set up for scaling up the number of qualified breastfeeding counselors in Afghanistan. A training-of-trainers (TOT) approach has been used at Kabul-area hospitals and is now being extended into the provinces. With UNICEF and WHO support, the MOPH's PND has trained 80 master trainers and 3,000 health workers in breastfeeding counseling in the country. The proportion of pregnant women who have been provided effective breastfeeding counseling is unknown.

A National Breastfeeding Communication Campaign was planned in 2008, spearheaded by UNICEF and implemented with the MOPH. After the 2009 World Breastfeeding Week (early August), the yearlong campaign was launched to promote improved breastfeeding practices (and

**Table 5.1    Current Initiatives Addressing IYCF in Afghanistan**

| Topic | Activity | Main partners |
|---|---|---|
| IYCF (general) | Information, education, and communication materials on IYCF | MOPH, NGOs, UNICEF, FAO, WHO, WFP |
| | Community-based growth monitoring and promotion | BASICS, MOPH, NGOs |
| | IMCI card for mothers on IYCF | BASICS, MOPH, NGOs, WHO |
| | Afghan Family Nutrition Guide | FAO, MAIL, MOPH, NGOs, |
| | Improved IYCF manual developed through formative research | FAO, MAIL, MOPH, UNICEF |
| | Introduction of nutrition education, including IYCF, in agriculture projects, literacy classes, and schools | FAO, MAIL, NGOs |
| | Positive Deviance/Health Nutrition Program | MOPH, Save the Children USA |
| Breastfeeding promotion | Baby-Friendly Hospital Initiative (limited) | MOPH, UNICEF |
| | Breastfeeding counseling: 3,000 counselors and 80 master trainers trained at national and provincial levels | MOPH, NGOs, UNICEF, WHO |
| | Relactation support for mothers in therapeutic feeding centers | Action Contre la Faim, MOPH |
| | Growth promotion (pilot) as maternal and child health nutrition platform | BASICS, MOPH, NGOs |
| | 40 provincial nutrition and reproductive health officers trained on maternal nutrition | MOPH, Tech-Serve |
| | Breastfeeding promotion campaign: <br> • Mass media campaign <br> • Celebration of Breastfeeding Week | MOPH, Ministry of Religious Affairs, Ministry of Women's Affairs, NGOs, UNICEF, WFP, WHO |
| | Afghanistan has adopted the International Code of Marketing of Breast Milk Substitutes | International Baby Food Action Network, International Code Documentation Centre, Ministry of Justice, MOPH, UNICEF |
| | South Asia Breastfeeding Forum, Kabul, 2006 | International Baby Food Action Network, Ministry of Foreign Affairs, MOPH, UNICEF, WHO, World Alliance for Breastfeeding Action |
| Complementary feeding | Development of Integrated Management of Childhood Illness complementary feeding card | MOPH, UNICEF, WHO |
| | Integration of cooking demonstrations in health, agriculture, and education projects (using manual) | FAO, MAIL, MOPH, NGOs |

*(continued)*

**Table 5.1    Current Initiatives Addressing IYCF in Afghanistan** *(continued)*

| Topic | Activity | Main partners |
|---|---|---|
| Micronutrients | Supplementation as part of BPHS and Essential Package of Hospital Services | MOPH, Micronutrient Initiative, UNICEF, NGOs |
| | Iodized salt; fortified flour (iron, zinc, vitamins A and B$_{12}$, folate) | Micronutrient Initiative, Ministry of Commerce, Ministry of Mines and Industry, MOPH, private sector, UNICEF, WFP |
| | Diet diversification: horticulture, poultry, livestock | MAIL |

*Source:* MOPH 2009.

---

**Box 5.5**

## IYCF Intervention Achievements, as of 2010

### Breastfeeding Promotion and Counseling

- Formative research on IYCF practices (Cornell University, MOPH, Save the Children, UNICEF)
- Development of breastfeeding counseling tools, and training of 80 master trainers and 3,000 total trainers at the health-facility level
- Introduction of relactation support as part of therapeutic feeding units (limited coverage)
- Adoption of the WHO's International Code of Marketing of Breast Milk Substitutes, endorsement of the code as a regulation under MOPH laws, and approval by the Ministry of Justice in 2008
- Introduction of the Baby-Friendly Hospital Initiative (limited success in four hospitals in Kabul)

### Complementary Feeding

- Formative research on complementary feeding practices through trials of improved practices (Cornell University, FAO, MAIL)
- Development of improved family and complementary feeding guidelines (manual produced by the MAIL and MOPH with FAO support: *Healthy Food, Happy Baby, Lively Family*)
- Introduction of training sessions in preparation of improved complementary foods in health, literacy, and agricultural projects (FAO, MAIL, UNICEF) (limited national coverage)

problem-solving techniques). Trained breastfeeding counselors (*khalas*) are paid to travel throughout the country during 2009 and 2010. Multimedia strategies (radio, television spots, and short films) are also being used, as well as distribution of posters and leaflets. The *khalas* will assist in developing community-level breastfeeding support groups, as recommended in the 10th step of the Baby-Friendly Hospital Initiative for ongoing support to mothers after the neonatal period. The Baby-Friendly Hospital Initiative has been attempted in four Kabul hospitals but has had limited success because of staff shortages, staff time, poor staff motivation, and monitoring challenges.

*Complementary feeding.* As noted earlier in this report, in the absence of a community nutrition worker, the health sector is currently limited in its capacity to provide IYCF trainings through BPHS facilities because time is rarely adequate for one-on-one behavior change counseling sessions with mothers (5–15 minutes is recommended) (Griffiths, Dickin, and Favin 1996). Alternative programs to support complementary feeding are therefore pursued jointly by the MOPH's PND and the MAIL's HED with support from FAO, UNICEF, the WHO, and the WFP. Jointly, these institutions have created training manuals that have been used in TOT sessions. Trainers (for example, MAIL provincial home economics officers) convene groups on behavior change communication and hands-on food preparation activities. National coverage of this program remains low. Existing staff members have capacity to scale up this program. Evaluations are done through qualitative focus groups.

The MAIL's HED, in partnership with MOPH provincial nutrition officers (PNOs) and FAO, trains women in five provinces in the preparation of appropriate complementary foods for children. These trainings are integrated into a range of community development projects (for example, food processing trainings) with literacy groups, producer groups, and other women's groups.

A manual for training caregivers on how to prepare culturally acceptable, improved complementary and family foods using local ingredients has been developed jointly by the MAIL, the MOPH, UNICEF, and FAO (see photo on next page).

The new WHO growth charts have been introduced in Afghanistan. Yet BPHS facilities generally do not perform growth promotion activities because of inability to regularly access mothers and inadequate staff time. Community-level structures are being used to pilot-test alternative approaches (box 5.6), and results have been encouraging.

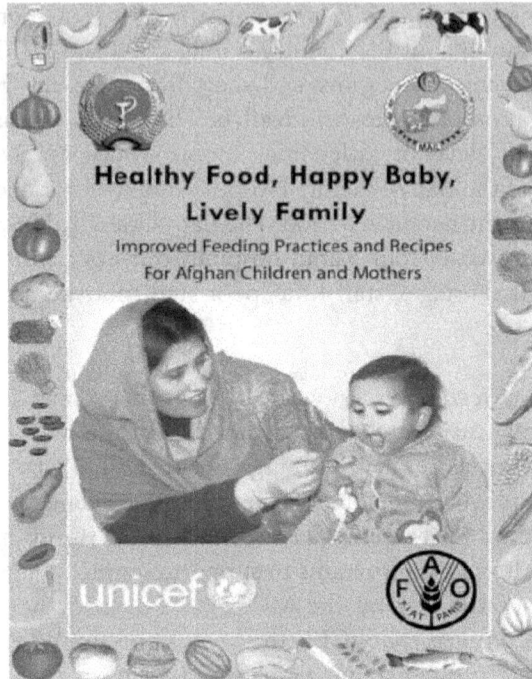

This manual for complementary feeding promotion is jointly produced by the MAIL's HED and the MOPH's PND. Photo courtesy of FAO-Afghanistan.

**Box 5.6**

## Community-Based Growth Promotion as a Platform for IYCF and Other Activities

Traditional, facility-based growth monitoring and promotion is unlikely to succeed in the Afghan context because of inadequate time for counseling, high female illiteracy rates, and women's irregular access to facilities (Levitt 2005). Therefore, a demonstration of a platform for disseminating information on optimal IYCF and maternal and child health is being carried out in one district in each of five provinces (Herat, Jowzjan, Takhar, Bamyan, and Kabul) with support from BASICS.

Growth promotion is part of the CHW job description, but CHWs have difficulty covering all households with a visit each month. In this new approach,

*(continued)*

**Box 5.6** *(continued)*

before getting to growth promotion, the CHW and the community health supervisor convince community leaders of the usefulness of establishing a family health action group (FHAG). Depending on the geographic area for which the CHW is responsible, the CHW will have 2 to 10 FHAGs.

The Growth Monitoring and Promotion program developed an approach to involve and link community-based growth monitoring promotion to CHWs without overloading them. The approach emphasizes weighing children in one central place with the help of the FHAGs. The CHW and the FHAG also conduct counseling of mothers. The growth-curve card has been made more user-friendly with a picture of the weighing scale face that uses the position of the scale's needle to determine the status of the child's weight gain or loss. A pictorial counseling card was also developed to conduct counseling targeted to mothers whose children have not gained the minimum adequate weight.

A female community member convenes the FHAG (10–15 houses) each month, focusing on those with children under two years of age (although no child younger than five years is turned away). Group members seek out mothers who do not appear for the sessions. The CHW joins the meeting and, with assistance of the group members, weighs the children and plots their weight gain (or lack thereof) on a simple pictorial chart (see appendix L). Given that many CHWs are illiterate, culturally appropriate pictorial materials have been developed and extensively pilot-tested. Educational materials allow guidance at different developmental stages for the child, based on the National IYCF Strategy. In-depth exploration of feeding practices is done for all children not gaining weight, and an agreement is made with the mother on how to modify behaviors. Children who do not gain weight for two successive months are referred to the nearest health facility. A group member conducts a follow-up visit. Children are checked for vaccination status and vitamin A supplementation. Sick children are managed according to the community-based IMCI protocol, which includes a household neonatal module. Hand washing with soap and use of insecticide-treated bed nets are encouraged. Pregnant women receive advice on prenatal care, birth planning and essential newborn care. Birth spacing is encouraged as a way of promoting healthy mothers and children.

The program is monitored every three months, and a final evaluation will occur after one year (July–September 2010). Positive initial response of the implementing NGOs has led the MOPH and USAID to integrate the approach in the new primary health care contracts of the BPHS implementers in the 13 USAID provinces.

A local business, Nutrition Zenda, has developed a fortified complementary food blend using local ingredients. The company (which evolved from a local NGO's "superflour" program for a maternal and child health project) is still small, is Kabul based, and would require support to scale up.

*Vitamin A supplementation.* Supplementation with vitamin A capsules can reduce mortality by up to 23 percent in Afghanistan (Bhutta and others 2008). In the absence of reliable prevalence data, existing information from varying sources (including the U5 mortality rate as a proxy indicator) has led to initiation of nationwide vitamin A campaigns twice a year for children (and postpartum women). These campaigns have been conducted with the National Immunization Days (NIDs) for polio. The NID campaign reported greater than 90 percent nationwide coverage for children 6 to 59 months old.

*Multiple micronutrient supplements for children.* The NIDs are not intended to continue indefinitely, so any future programs must be fully functional before discontinuation of the NIDs. The Micronutrient Initiative (MI) has funds for a pilot program to explore longer-term vitamin A strategies outside the NIDs, to help prepare Afghanistan for eventual phaseout of that delivery platform.

Use of micronutrient powders has been shown to reduce anemia risk in children 6 to 24 months old by 21 percent (Bhutta and others 2008). In many countries, home-based multiple micronutrient powders (such as Sprinkles and Anuka) are available through public systems, through the private sector, or through public-private partnerships. These powders are added to the child's food just before eating. They are commonly provided as a single-serving sachet, with instructions for daily use over a set period of time. According to the U.S. Centers for Disease Control and Prevention, social marketing of Sprinkles in Kenya has led to over 50 percent coverage.[1] Anecdotal reports of offering Sprinkles to Afghan households revealed high levels of interest in this type of product for improving child nutrition.[2] As stated in the 2009 national micronutrient strategy, Afghanistan is going to explore the feasibility of multiple micronutrient powders through a market study. MI is currently supporting a pilot free distribution of micronutrient powders in high-burden provinces.

*Vitamin C.* The PND and UNICEF have instituted a strategy to avert outbreaks of scurvy. Preventive vitamin C doses are to be administered during two or three winter months to communities deemed to be at high risk. UNICEF has provided support for this preventive supplementation intervention, distributing the supplements in advance of winter. A multiple micronutrient powder strategy could also effectively address concerns about vitamin C deficiency.

***Zinc and diarrhea control.*** The revised BPHS includes zinc along with oral rehydration solution for the control of diarrheal diseases. Currently, zinc supplements have 50 percent coverage in provinces supported by USAID (with UNICEF and Tech-Serve). Scale-up is urgently needed in the remaining provinces supported by the World Bank and the European Commission.

***Anemia prevention activities.*** Various interventions are included in the BPHS to reduce anemia risk. The IMCI program screens children for anemia and provides treatment (liquid iron supplement). No coverage data were identified. Malaria control activities are also receiving strong support. Deworming medications are provided free through the BPHS, but no data are available on prevalence of worm infections or coverage of preschool children.

***Treatment of acute undernutrition.*** Because levels of acute undernutrition in U5 children are generally below 10 percent, and because the health system has increased in reach and capacity, the largely NGO-run therapeutic feeding centers have been transferred over to government-run hospital-based care. Operation of hospital-based therapeutic feeding units (TFUs) is now a component in the MOPH's Essential Package of Hospital Services. With UNICEF and WHO support, PNOs are responsible for oversight of the 38 TFUs in provincial and district hospitals. Community-Based Management of Acute Malnutrition (CMAM) was being piloted and considered for inclusion in national policy during the time of this review.

In a focus group of 15 PNOs from across Afghanistan,[3] the following constraints were identified and some recommendations offered to enhance facility-based program effectiveness:

- *Families have low levels of nutrition awareness.* Nutrition promotion must be incorporated into programming to decrease the likelihood that children will relapse and to prevent acute undernutrition in other children in the household.

- *Bed capacity is low, and often multiple children are kept in one bed.* For example, in Kunar province, the TFU has eight beds. In summer and fall, occupancy can be as high as 30 to 40 children.
- *TFUs do not have enough staff for the work required.* One or two staff persons are responsible for operating the TFU. Because the workload is greater than for other hospital departments and no added incentive or support is provided to staff, the TFU is the least desired post in the hospital. Many nurses are not willing to work there unless they can have higher salaries because of the difficulty of the work. PNOs request four nurses and one doctor per TFU.
- *Resources are inadequate for meeting treatment needs.* Medicines often run out by the middle of the month, and time for procurement leads to delays in replenishing supply in time for proper care.
- *Space allocated to some TFUs violates protocols.* Some TFUs lack a stock room for supplies. All activities are performed in the same room (which does *not* meet the code).
- *Many families will not come to TFUs.* Because of cultural constraints on women being away from home in general, and particularly overnight, TFUs are not used as fully as they could be.
- *PNOs are constrained in their ability to monitor TFUs outside the provincial capital.* No transportation is provided, and no budget has been allocated for transportation. PNOs are requested to partner with other departments or organizations that have vehicles. Vehicle availability is limited.

In addition to the TFUs, the community-based care models are being explored. The Public Nutrition Strategy for 2009–13 has determined that supplementary feeding programs will be used when global acute malnutrition or wasting is greater than 10 percent (targeted feeding) and when global acute malnutrition is greater than 15 percent (blanket feeding). Current demonstration projects include the following:

- In partnership with BPHS NGOs, community-based management of severe acute undernutrition has been established in nine provinces and will be scaled up in three more provinces (with UNICEF and WHO support). Coverage remains limited.
- As part of the CMAM pilot started in the first half of 2009, supplementary feeding programs were established. (Supplementary feeding centers had previously been implemented in 2002 and 2003, not as part of CMAM but with the WFP.) The CMAM Task Force is finalizing the

revised CMAM guideline for Afghanistan under which the whole CMAM package will be implemented as a package through the BPHS.

*Gaps and opportunities related to infant and young child nutrition.* Several challenges remain:

- Breastfeeding practices are not adequate during the first two years. Breastfeeding counselors are being trained in increasing numbers in the BPHS system. Community platforms are also being explored for broader IYCF work inclusive of breastfeeding promotion (for example, the BASICS pilot). A campaign held during 2009 to 2010 was supported largely by UNICEF.
- The MAIL's HED has budgets at national and provincial levels for promotion of optimal complementary feeding practices in five provinces. More than 20 trainers have been trained and are available to work in 12 more provinces. Activities are conducted in five provinces through FAO funding. Officers in the existing provinces have time to scale up.
- Support is required for design and printing of HED materials for use at the community level. Existing materials are designed for trainers.
- Community platforms are needed for promoting complementary feeding. The BASICS demonstration project may prove an effective method, using CHWs and family health action groups appropriate to the Afghan context (see box 5.6). A cadre of community nutrition workers may also need to be developed, initially on a pilot scale.
- Local producers with large-scale capacity to produce fortified complementary foods are lacking. One small producer (Nutrition Zenda) exists, which could increase capacity if resources were available to assist with business development. Developing a sustainable business model will be important. The product (see accompanying photo) may reach only urban and peri-urban areas in the near term unless improved distribution and pricing (for example, through a public-private partnership arrangement) are achieved to increase availability and economic access for a wider rural market.
- A strategy for vitamin A supplementation outside of the NIDs needs to be developed. Given the highly cost-effective platform provided by the NIDs, the vitamin A distribution should not be delinked from the NIDs until the latter phase out.
- Zinc supplementation (with oral rehydration solution) for the treatment of diarrhea should be scaled up within the BPHS in accordance with the revised policy.

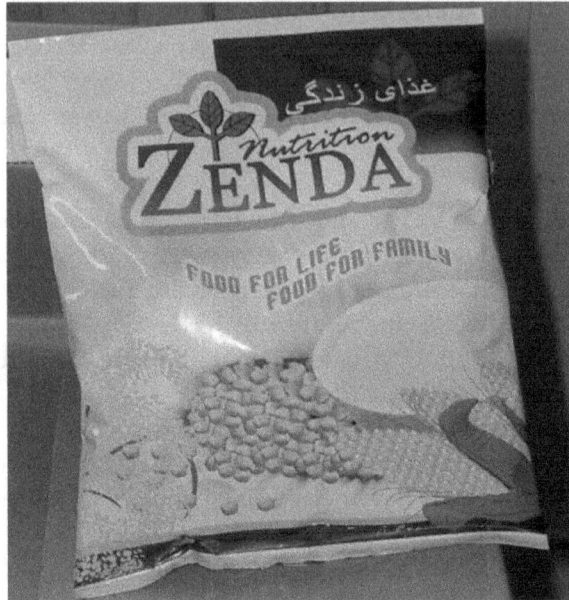

Nutrition Zenda is a fortified
complementary food currently
produced by a small business in Kabul.
Photo courtesy of Emily Levitt.

- Coverage of deworming for pregnant women and preschool children should be increased to reduce risk of anemia.
- Multiple micronutrient powders may be an effective intervention to address high rates of childhood anemia and other micronutrient deficiencies such as vitamin C in Afghanistan. A market study is needed to determine the feasibility of this intervention and marketing and promotional strategies.
- Hand-washing promotion should continue, given the 30 percent reduction in diarrhea risk.

### Food Fortification
Food fortification includes fortification of flour, salt, and oil and ghee.

*Flour fortification.* Approximately 74 percent of the Afghan population is rural, and the majority of rural households (81 percent) use flour milled locally by small village mills (MOPH and others 2009). By contrast, among the urban population of the country, 73 percent of households reported buying flour from the market (figure 5.2). Currently, eight

**Figure 5.2    Flour Purchasing Behavior among Households with Flour Available, 2004**

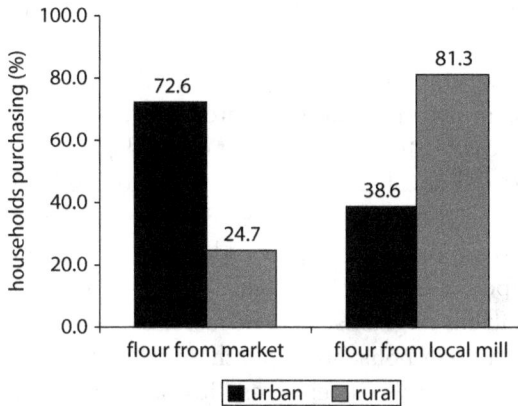

*Source:* MOPH and others 2009.

private industrial flour mills operate in Afghanistan. The WFP has supported the voluntary installation of microfeeders in these mills, which fortify flour with iron, zinc, vitamin $B_{12}$, vitamin A, and folic acid. The mills receive the fortificant premix through MI funding. Current urban coverage of fortified wheat flour is estimated to be only about 8 percent, and some 60 percent of people buying the flour are from the poorest customer group.

*Universal salt iodization and double-fortified salt.* Consumption of iodized salt is important for maternal nutritional well-being and for prevention of mental impairment in a developing unborn child and prevention of stillbirths. A national universal salt iodization campaign began in 2003 to address the problem of endemic iodine deficiency. This program is supported at the highest levels of government. President Hamid Karzai has issued a decree that all Afghan households should use iodized salt. Twenty-five salt factories in Afghanistan now fortify salt from domestic sources, enabling the country to be self-sufficient in salt. An Afghan salt producers association exists and is committed to manufacturing adequately iodized salt, provided its members can procure sufficient good-quality raw salt at a reasonable price. Fortificants are currently provided by MI and UNICEF, but a sustainable strategy does not yet exist. The MOPH's PND monitors the factories every two months and collaborates closely with MI on program delivery and monitoring issues. A school-based monitoring system run by the MOPH's PND and UNICEF monitors samples of household salt. Double fortification of salt with iron as well as iodine will require additional support and is being explored by MI, the MOPH, and UNICEF, in light of successes in India.

Iodized salt coverage is currently estimated at 50 percent. However, domestic salt is mined using crude approaches leading to contamination with mud and possibly heavy metals (for example, lead). Consumers view the darker (iodized and local) salt as "dirty" and prefer to purchase salt smuggled from neighboring countries. Because salt processors have no legal recourse to import rock salt, the industry is facing serious challenges. MI has developed a funding proposal for a salt purification facility to clean Afghan salt for Afghanistan's salt factories.

Virtually all Afghan households purchase salt (99.5 percent). Regional differences in iodized salt use exist, as illustrated in figure 5.3. The male head of household typically determines the type of salt acquired (table 5.2). These data suggest that communication or social marketing efforts related to use of iodized salt by Afghan households should especially target males.

Men and women differed in their awareness about the importance of consuming iodized salt. Among both genders, those who were literate and those with any schooling were significantly more likely to have heard of iodized salt than were those who were illiterate or had no schooling ($p < 0.05$).

**Figure 5.3    Household Coverage of Iodized Salt in Survey Clusters in Kabul and in Clusters in Rest of the Country, 2004**

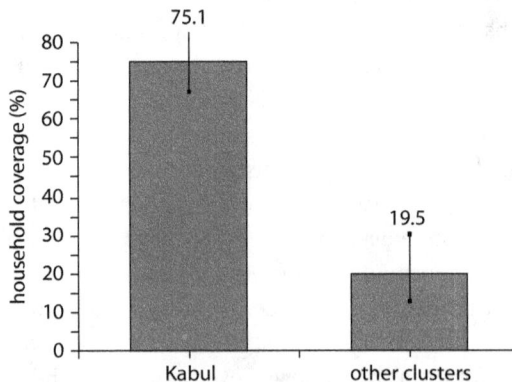

*Source:* MOPH and others 2009.

**Table 5.2    Proportion of Households Purchasing Salt and the Individual Who Usually Decides on the Type of Salt to Purchase, 2004**

| Household characteristics | Percent |
|---|---|
| Household buys salt | |
| Yes | 99.5 |
| Who most often decides which type of salt to buy? | |
| Male head of household | 87.3 |
| Other adult male | 8.1 |
| Female head of household | 3.0 |
| Other adult female | 0.2 |
| Child | 0.6 |
| Shopkeeper | 0.5 |
| Other | 0.1 |

Source: MOPH and others 2009.

*Oil and ghee fortification with vitamin A.* In the national micronutrient strategy (MOPH 2009), plans exist to explore fortification of both cooking oil and ghee with vitamin A. The 2004 National Nutrition Survey found that cooking oil (like salt) was largely acquired at markets and purchased by men. Nearly 90 percent of the cooking oil and ghee purchased was labeled as vitamin A fortified, but tests showed that only 10 percent of 40 tested samples were actually fortified.

*Gaps and opportunities related to food fortification.* Food fortification presents a number of challenges and opportunities:

- The government of Afghanistan has not issued national flour fortification standards (for example, WHO's recommendations of iron, folate, zinc, vitamin $B_{12}$, and vitamin A). The type of fortification premix varies depending on what development partners provide.
- Reaching rural areas with fortified flour has been a challenge; therefore, double-fortified salt is a preferred strategy for reaching rural populations with an iron-fortified staple food.
- More technical and financial assistance is needed for industrial flour mills to properly operate fortification equipment (microfeeders). Partial support exists from the WFP and MI.
- Quality control capacity is weak in flour mills, and national capacity to perform legal quality control checks on fortified flour is lacking. MI is working with the MOPH to increase the latter's capacity to monitor mills.

- An industry association for private flour millers, as occurs in other countries, does not yet exist, which complicates public-private sector relations.
- Flour imports are not generally fortified, and importers are unaware of the importance of fortified flour. MI had been fortifying flour in Pakistan for export to Afghanistan until Pakistan banned the export of wheat flour following the food price crisis. No national regulation mandates that imported flour be fortified, even though all countries exporting to Afghanistan have the capacity to fortify such flour.
- No regular monitoring system is in effect to determine household coverage of fortified flour use. Coordination with the MRRD's NRVA or MAIL's Food Security Surveillance initiative should be considered. The Afghanistan National Standards Authority (ANSA) could also be involved with enforcement but would need capacity-building support to do so.
- A salt purification facility is urgently needed for decontaminating domestic salt sources and providing an acceptable, safe source for consumers. This salt purification facility could also serve as the production site for double-fortified salt.
- Subsequent to improvements in domestic salt quality, a national information, education, and communication campaign (especially through the media and health services) will be required to restore consumer confidence in domestic salt.
- Strategies are needed to increase access to and use of iodized salt outside of Kabul. Promotion of the benefits of iodized salt should be focused especially on men, who predominantly purchase salt for the household.
- Capacity building may be needed for the domestic private sector if vitamin A fortification of local oils and ghee is feasible. More often, oil and ghee are imported, and capacity building will be required for importers to appropriately source fortified products. Quality control is needed to identify cooking oil and ghee falsely labeled as vitamin A fortified. ANSA is not a strong institution and is constrained by private sector interests pressuring authorities to limit regulation.

## Pillar 4: Determinants of Undernutrition Are Addressed through Multisectoral Approaches

Although the government of Afghanistan has instituted policies to address the underlying causes of undernutrition, significant gaps in program coverage remain. Food security, health and health services, health environment, and care for women and children would be the main interventions within this pillar. Nutrition promotion to the general public could also be included. Many interventions related to health and care of women and children were covered under Pillar 3.

### Food Security Interventions

Food security interventions include a number of programs, from surveillance to availability to safety and quality control initiatives.

*Food security surveillance.* Since 2002, a few food security surveillance and early-warning initiatives have been developed in Afghanistan. They provide data on food prices, agricultural production, livelihood strategies, and agriculture-related weather. These systems are supported by various institutions (FAO, the MAIL, USAID's Agromet, USAID's Famine Early Warning Systems Network, and the WFP's Vulnerability Assistance Mapping). Despite these varied activities, some major challenges exist to food security surveillance. These initiatives are poorly coordinated or integrated, large data collection efforts result in extensive delays, and data quality varies. The MAIL has prepared a concept note on strengthening integrated food security surveillance as a component of its change management program. Whereas the MAIL follows food security indicators throughout the year, the MRRD's NRVA is a resource for monitoring household-level food security trends on a periodic basis (generally every other year).

Many gaps and opportunities exist related to food security surveillance:

- Afghanistan lacks an effective, centralized food security surveillance system that provides timely and accurate information essential to inform development planning and emergency interventions.
- Institutions with existing surveillance systems have agreed to work together to improve coordination of current food security surveillance activities. The MAIL requires technical assistance to strengthen its Statistics Department, to support interagency coordination, and to ensure that concrete results are generated. It has prepared a concept note with a detailed plan for how to address this gap.

*Food availability.* Improving food availability—both domestic production and food importation—is the responsibility of various government ministries. Implicated sectors include agriculture, rural development, commerce, energy, and water, among others. Current activities within the agriculture sector include improved seeds (through seed production enterprises), plant protection and integrated pest management, emergency tools and seed distribution, and emergency food aid distribution. Although funding for such activities is forthcoming from various bilateral agencies and development partners, continued advocacy is needed for agricultural production that supports *household* food security within the country. Too frequently, agriculture is viewed only through a commercial, income-generating lens. Household food security indicators are rarely included as output measures in current agricultural projects. For example, the World Bank–funded Horticulture and Livestock Project (HLP) focuses impact assessments on income generation. Two livestock programs are described later in this section; however, varied horticulture producer groups are open to nutrition promotion supported by the HLP Farmer Organizations Department.

As with food security, the gaps and opportunities related to general food availability are numerous:

- Advocacy at high levels is needed in the agriculture sector (specifically, the MAIL) to include impact indicators on child nutritional status and household food security of current MAIL programs, including the HLP. This inclusion is justified given that improved household food security is one of the ultimate goals of the MAIL's National Agriculture Development Framework.
- Diet diversity, food frequency, and caloric consumption measurements exist and have been included in national surveys such as the NRVA. Technical staff members in the MOPH's PND, the MAIL's HED, FAO, and the WFP are available to assist with indicator selection.
- The HLP Farmer Organizations Department has offered its more than 100 women's farmer groups and other men's farmer groups as educational platforms. The HLP staff proposed forming a committee to design a nutrition promotion curriculum. The HLP staff welcomed the MAIL's HED officers as trainers and suggested that topics be coordinated with the seasonal agricultural calendar.

FAO's experience in Afghanistan and studies elsewhere have shown that a combined (packaged) approach is most effective with agriculture-nutrition projects in achieving changes in household nutrition practices (see box 5.7). This success has been attributed to investing in multiple forms of human capital (Berti, Krasevec, and FitzGerald 2004).

**Box 5.7**

## Using a Packaged Approach to Interventions

Although no quantitative evaluations have been conducted, FAO reports qualita-tive evidence from focus groups that a packaged approach reinforces single inter-ventions and catalyzes household-level behavior change. The existing package used in communities with FAO and NGO support for the MAIL's HED includes

- Nutrition promotion through platforms of food processing, storage, and income-generation activities, including family food options to diversify house-hold diets
- Instruction through women's groups on improved complementary feeding
- School-based nutrition promotion

These initial findings are consistent with a recent review of nutrition-agriculture linked interventions (Berti, Krasevec, and FitzGerald 2004), which found that investments in different types of capital in the same community are more likely than any one intervention to result in positive nutritional outcomes. Intervention packages incorporating nutrition education and a focus on women are more likely to lead to positive nutritional outcomes than those with other program components. To be effective, nutrition promotion in food insecure populations may require a food supplement or conditional cash transfer scheme (Bhutta and others 2008). However, in unstable societies, the logistics of program delivery must be considered. Thus, in Afghanistan, promoting community-based food security programs with nutrition promotion may be more worthwhile because these interventions teach life skills for longer-term poverty alleviation.

Afghanistan currently has several agriculture programs that could have a nutritional effect, but these programs are operating at a limited scale. Those with the possibility of scaling up (and being included in a pack-age with nutrition promotion activities by the MAIL's HED) are described in the following sections.

*HLP Backyard Poultry Project.* The MAIL works with FAO (its World Bank–funded implementing partner) to run a three-year US$5 million poultry project in 10 provinces (begun in 2009). The objectives of the project are to improve household nutrition and economic status. Data from 2003 show that Afghanistan imports US$29 million of eggs per year and US$90 million of chicken, fed by strong domestic demand for these commodities. In the project's first year, 10 districts were selected per each of the 10 provinces for intervention (total 100 districts). The program is targeting 1,000 vulnerable women in each district (total 100,000 women). The project is scheduled to scale up to another 100,000 women in 2010, doubling the coverage (total 200,000 in program).

Opportunities for nutrition with the HLP Backyard Poultry Project include the following:

- *Nutrition promotion.* The project currently has no direct nutrition promotion component. Eggs and chicken both provide significant sources of nutrients for households. FAO and other partner institutions have studied local beliefs about these foods, and culturally appropriate nutrition promotion messages exist (see appendix C). The poultry project provides an excellent, available platform for nutrition promotion.
- *Nutrition indicators.* The project measures only household income as an outcome of the program and does not currently include any measures of effects on household consumption patterns. Advocacy and technical support are needed for inclusion of nutrition-related indicators in this project, particularly for women and children. Linking support to use of nutrition indicators should be considered.

*HLP Integrated Dairy Schemes Project.* The MAIL works with GRM International to implement the dairy component of the World Bank–funded HLP. This project component builds on several earlier dairy programs operated by FAO, among others. The program targets women and is designed around local dairy cooperatives to improve household food security and income. Women are particularly involved with dairy work because they milk and care for the cows. The program is currently designed to cover three provinces to the north of Kabul (Kabul, Parwan, and Kapisa). The original budget was approximately US$4.8 million (building cost for plant not included).

Opportunities for nutrition through the dairy project:

- *Nutrition promotion.* The project currently has no direct nutrition promotion component. Dairy products and beef from male calves have the potential to provide significant sources of nutrients for households. FAO and other partner institutions have studied local beliefs about these foods, and culturally appropriate nutrition promotion messages exist (see appendix C). The dairy project provides an excellent available platform for nutrition promotion.

- *Nutrition indicators.* The project measures only household income as an outcome of the program and does not currently include any measures of effects on household consumption patterns. Advocacy and technical support are needed for inclusion of nutrition-related indicators in this project, particularly for women and children.

*Project promoting improved household-level food processing, preservation, and storage.* With support from FAO and the United Nations Industrial Development Organization (UNIDO), the HED works to scale up a project to promote nutrition in vulnerable rural households in the context of education about food processing, preservation, and storage. The project helps address the gap in food security during winter months by providing nutritious foods during the vulnerable season as well as a source of additional household income. Foods preserved or sold for additional income include jams, juice, pickled vegetables, tomato paste, ketchup, and vinegar. The project operates in five provinces through various community-level platforms: mothers' and women's groups, literacy groups, producer groups, and self-help groups. HED officers conduct TOTs with schoolteachers, literacy teachers, government workers, youth clubs, and other local leaders. The HED provides the materials necessary for the training (see photo on next page).

Gaps and opportunities related to the HED food processing project include the following:

- The HED has staff members in 17 provinces, but its budget limits their activities to 5 provinces. The project is currently supported as one component of a broader FAO grant from the German government that ends after 2010.

- This program provides an available, easily scalable platform for reaching vulnerable women with nutrition promotion messages. For example, the project could be expanded to additional women's groups in the HLP and the National Solidarity Program (NSP). Various studies have shown that approaches emphasizing home production of nutrient-rich foods do not result in significant nutritional improvements unless they are complemented by nutrition promotion activities (Brun, Reynaud, and Chevassus-Agnes 1989; English and Badcock 1998; Kennedy and Alderman 1987; Marsh 1998). This program provides knowledge

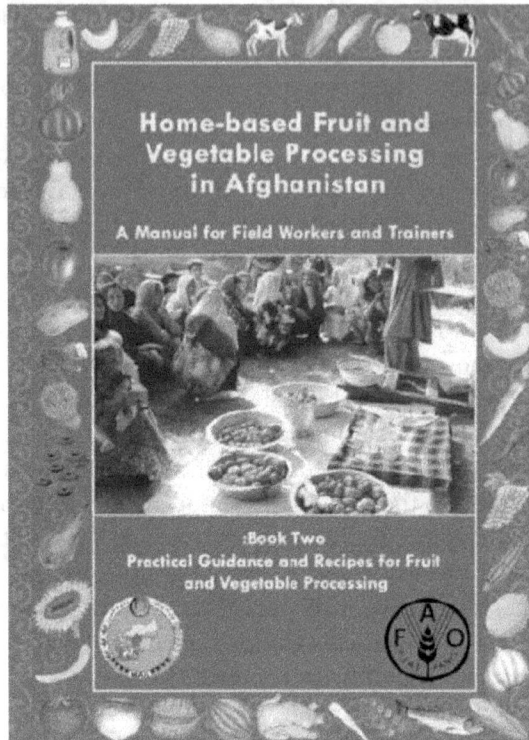

This manual on food processing and
preservation is produced by the MAIL's HED
and FAO. Photo courtesy of FAO-Afghanistan.

and skills for improving household food security (reducing postharvest losses) as well as a source of income for increasing profit margins on raw agricultural products through value-added food processing. The project is currently not achieving very significant national coverage.

*School-Based Nutrition Program.*  With funding provided through FAO, the MAIL's HED is currently scaling up a nutrition promotion program that reaches primary and secondary school students (grades 1–12) in seven provinces. This program brings back to Afghanistan life-skills training traditionally incorporated into the Afghan public school curriculum but interrupted during the war years. Current coverage is 155 schools, and each school is responsible for training 5 other schools in the surrounding area. Support for this program from community leaders and elders is very high (even nostalgic), and nonparticipating schools frequently request initiation of the program.

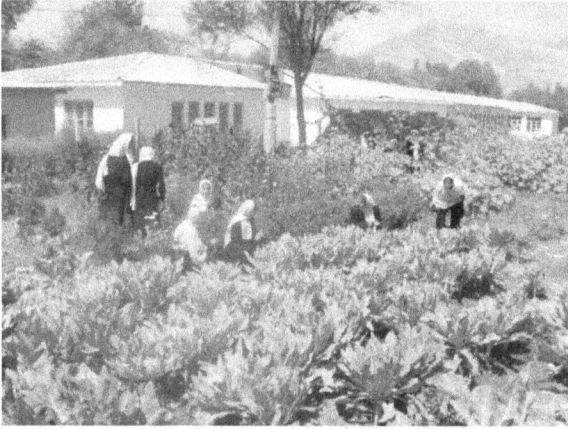

The MAIL's School-Based Nutrition Program teaches
girls (and boys) using gardens as an educational
platform. Photo courtesy of FAO-Afghanistan.

Teachers from each school are trained in key nutrition messages linked with a school garden. Five minutes are devoted to promoting key nutrition messages every day of the school year, a concession given the shortened school time available for instruction (in some cases, two hours per student cohort). Teachers instruct students how to plant and care for the garden and how to harvest, process, and consume different types of vegetables and legumes (see accompanying photo). This project is implemented in collaboration with the Ministry of Education, the MOPH, and the Ministry of Youth Affairs. The Healthy Schools Initiative (1,000 schools) and National Youth Program (joint UN programs) partner with this program and are exploring means to scale up.

Opportunities related to the School-Based Nutrition Program are as follows:

- Platforms for reaching girls are few before they are engaged or married and become pregnant. Recent figures show over half of girls are married by age 17 (CSO 2009). The program is a platform that reaches girls with key individual and family nutrition messages. Women are the main food preparers for the household. Trainers confirmed that current curriculum could be expanded to highlight the importance of nutrition through the life course. Curriculum for girls could incorporate nutrition prior to pregnancy, during pregnancy, and lactation as well as IYCF. Boys and girls typically attend school at different times of day, thus facilitating gender-specific discussions such as nutrition for prepregnant, pregnant, and lactating women. The current training program on nutrition for the CHWs could be adapted for use in schools.

- Boys also are important targets because men primarily do the shopping and have influence over household behaviors, including food consumption. Given that marriage is a near-universal phenomenon in Afghanistan, male children will need to be aware of the nutritional needs of all household members as future providers. Impact evaluations are needed to assess changes in knowledge, attitudes, and practices among children in participating schools and the degree to which these programs influence household practices.

***Food hygiene, food safety, and quality control.*** The MOPH, the MAIL, the Ministry of Commerce, and FAO work on improving food hygiene (proper care and use), food safety, and quality control. The Ministry of Commerce has established ANSA for quality control of various products, including foods, with support from UNIDO. ANSA currently has limited implementation capacity and is pressured by commercial interests seeking to avoid regulation; however, it is an important component of Afghanistan's nutrition system because ANSA should perform quality control tests on fortified foods. Currently, many foods labeled as fortified are not actually fortified (MOPH and others 2009). Reportedly, this situation is in part caused by the availability of certain types of (marked) containers and lack of regulation and enforcement of Afghan imports.

Various gaps and opportunities exist in this area:

- Infectious diseases arising from poor food hygiene, inadequate food safety, and lack of quality control contribute to the very high levels of diarrhea and other infections in Afghan children and adults. These diseases are preventable through simple interventions (for example, soaking fruit and vegetables in water with chlorine, iodine, or potassium permanganate) and basic practices related to food handling. Sanitizing products are available at low cost in the local markets, but awareness about their use is limited.

- The Healthy Schools Initiative may be a useful partner for increasing public awareness, because the sole nutrition message taught through government schools has pertained to avoiding eating leftover foods (because of the inadequate refrigeration). Incorporating a few additional messages into this curriculum should be easy and yield results.

Likewise, the School-Based Nutrition Program run by the MAIL's HED could include these messages as a teaching point.

- ANSA is a new entity that needs significant support to adequately monitor foods and to enforce government regulations pertaining to foods, such as verifying fortification levels. Sufficient support will be required for the staff of this agency to counter the bribes offered by commercial entities trying to avoid regulation.

*Other relevant agriculture and rural development activities.*  Other technical agency partners are working to improve animal health services (the European Union and USAID); perennial horticulture development (the European Union, USAID, and the World Bank); natural resource management; and commercial agriculture development. In addition, many NGOs are actively engaged in integrated agricultural development at community level, introducing improved agricultural and natural resource management techniques as part of broader development activities, namely the MRRD's NSP. The Ministry of Energy and Water (with support from FAO and the World Bank, the European Union, the Asian Development Bank, and USAID) implements large-scale irrigation projects that have a key effect on food production and food security. Varied MRRD programs listed in table 4.1 in chapter 4 also make an essential contribution to food security and sustainable livelihoods. At the moment, these projects are fragmented and have not yet been brought into a coordinated national action plan.

*Opportunities to partner with other sectors to improve food security.*  Although the following programs do not currently include human nutrition promotion elements, each expressed interest in being a platform for such activities:

- The NSP welcomes nutrition promotion activities through its network of more than 22,000 community development committees (CDCs). It aims to scale up to another 9,000 CDCs in the next project cycle, which should complete country coverage.
- Senior advisers to the MAIL minister recommended using mobile veterinary unit technicians as conduits of nutrition information to the community. They recommended providing pamphlets with basic nutrition messages to the mobile veterinary unit offices for distribution. Basic training in the use of these materials would be useful. The HED staff could develop these pamphlets with technical support from FAO and the MOPH's PND.

## Health, Health Services, and Health Environment

In addition to providing many of the direct nutrition interventions, the health sector is involved in activities to tackle disease-related causes of undernutrition. This section emphasizes the programs targeted at reducing infectious diseases and the services relevant to improving the quality of the health environment (clean drinking water and improved sanitation).

*Activities to reduce infectious diseases.* The BPHS includes a number of activities targeted at reducing infectious diseases, a key contributing cause to chronic and acute undernutrition, as well as vitamin and mineral deficiencies. Several development partners, including the European Commission, USAID, and the World Bank, strongly support primary health care in Afghanistan. Several programs relevant to nutrition are described under Pillar 3.

Another program is the Expanded Programme on Immunization. WHO recommends the full immunization of children 12 to 23 months of age for tuberculosis (Bacillus Calmette-Guérin tuberculosis vaccine); polio (oral polio vaccine type 3); diphtheria, pertussis, and tetanus (three doses of the diphtheria, pertussis, and tetanus vaccine); and measles. According to the NRVA 2007/08, national coverage with full immunization is low, at 37 percent, and 15 percent of children have never been immunized. Urban children had higher rates of immunization than did rural children. The lowest rates were found among the children of *Kuchi* households (see figure 5.4). Higher education of the mother was positively related to her child's positive immunization status (CSO 2009).

A semi-annual campaign (NIDs for polio eradication) includes vitamin A supplementation. Apart from campaigns, routine visits are made at the recommendation of the CHW to comply with WHO's Expanded Programme on Immunization.

In addition, the MOPH runs multiple disease reduction programs. The IMCI program is the main initiative for addressing diseases in children. National programs also cover tuberculosis control and HIV/AIDS risk reduction and treatment. General health service access and use are the predominant health systems concerns, as noted in chapter 3.

Gaps and opportunities related to disease control programs include the following:

• Disease control through government services in insecure areas is difficult.

**Figure 5.4    Data on Vaccination Coverage for Children, by Residence, 2007/08**

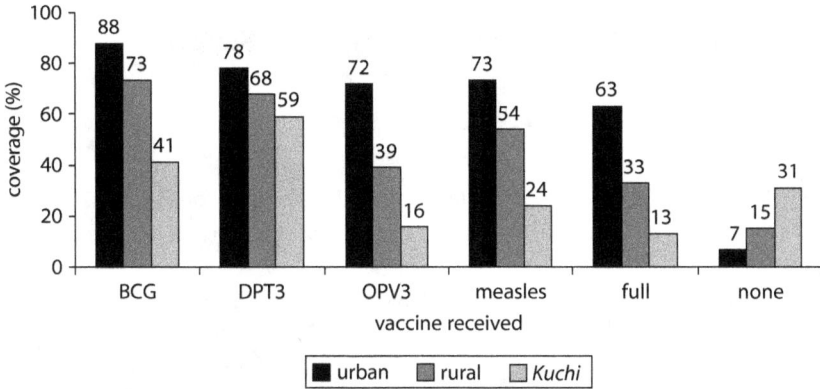

*Source:* CSO 2009.
*Note:* BCG = Bacillus Calmette-Guérin tuberculosis vaccine; DPT3 = three doses of the diphtheria, pertussis, and tetanus vaccine, which is required for complete coverage; OPV3 = oral polio vaccine type 3.

- Improved immunization coverage, particularly at the recommended times for infants, is still too low.
- A wider support system is needed for community health activities. CHWs have many tasks already. The family health action groups and community health *shura*s (councils) have been piloted in some provinces as a strategy to provide added support to the CHWs.

***Water and sanitation activities.*** Principles of the national policy on water supply and sanitation are listed in box 5.8. The MRRD supports two activities to improve access to water and sanitation.

*Rural Water, Sanitation, and Irrigation Program.* Clean drinking water interventions for rural areas are supported by MRRD's Department of Water, Sanitation, and Irrigation under the Rural Water, Sanitation, and Irrigation Program (RuWatSIP). RuWatSIP directly supports activities in 24 of 34 provinces and provides a package of services to communities that solicit support. The package includes a safe drinking water supply, construction of demonstration latrines, and hygiene messages. Materials have been developed for education components that are appropriate for illiterate audiences. RuWatSIP also supports the NSP's community development committees, which themselves present requests for specific services to the MRRD. These requests do not necessarily include the whole RuWatSIP package.

**Box 5.8**

## Principles of the National Policy on Water Supply and Sanitation

- Reduce the average time taken to fetch water from four hours to one hour (round trip).
- Provide basic service to all, defined as 25 liters per person per day or one water point from any type of water supply source for every 25 families or 175 individuals.
- Integrate programs for safe water supply, hygiene education, and demonstration latrines.
- Provide advocacy and support for simple technologies that can be operated and maintained with the community-level capacities.

*Source:* Reji 2007.

An evaluation of RuWatSIP activities occurred in 2007 (Reji 2007). According to a representative, random sample of beneficiaries, 83 percent of men and 96 percent of women reported a major reduction in prevalence of waterborne diseases, especially among children. Local health authorities corroborated these reports. Likewise from this study, where the package approach was implemented, 76 percent of men and 78 percent of women stated that changes in personal hygiene behavior had occurred. Men and women also noted that these behavior changes were the cumulative effect of various promotional activities, including those of the CHWs trained by provincial health departments and NGOs. Improved water sources closer to communities have also reportedly decreased the workload of women and children, who are typically responsible for collecting water for domestic uses.

The benefits for improved nutrition are multiple—decreasing excessive caloric expenditure for water collection and increasing the caregiving capacity for infants and young children. Seventy-three percent of women stated that they used the time saved for improved care of their families and gave greater attention to their infants. The remaining 23 percent stated that they used the time for farming activities or other income-generating work. Moreover, 75 percent of women surveyed reported increased school attendance of children. Focus groups with children confirmed this outcome: children stated they could more easily arrive at school on time because less time was required for early-morning water retrieval. The relationship between girls' obtaining education and improved nutrition practices has been widely acknowledged.

Although current funding is US$25 million, current community requests for support from RuWatSIP total US$85 million, including requests for the package of interventions and NSP requests for specific components. Given the low coverage rates of access to safe water and of use of improved sanitation facilities and hygiene practices, scaling up of the RuWatSIP should be given priority.

The following gaps and opportunities exist:

- Support is requested that is not tied to a specific province. Such support can meet demands coming from communities in *any* province (if current demand exceeds the budget for that province), including provinces that have no earmarked funding.
- Support for additional staff will be required to expedite the scale-up of activities.
- Maternal underweight could be related to travel distance required to obtain water; hence, targeting water projects to areas with a high prevalence of maternal underweight (low body mass index) should be considered.

*MRRD's NSP Program.* As previously noted, the MRRD's NSP also contributes to water and sanitation activities. According to MRRD authorities, the top request from the 22,000-plus communities participating in the NSP is for interventions to support safe drinking water.[4] Another 9,000 communities will be added to the NSP in the next program cycle. The CDCs are awarded block grants to use as they choose. MRRD authorities remarked that communities currently without safe drinking water almost always request this intervention first. When communities have safe water, focus shifts to other livelihood-related interventions (for example, irrigation canals, roads, and retaining walls). The NSP is therefore a critical vehicle for any strategy aimed at increasing access to improved water and sanitation facilities.

Through the NSP, the MRRD aims to reach 15 million rural people with access to safe drinking water and sanitation facilities by 2013. Also, the MRRD has offered the CDCs as a platform for other health or nutrition promotion. Officials cited the example of UNICEF, which has used the CDCs for promoting various public health messages. Figure 5.5 shows the coverage and gap in coverage for safe water in rural areas as of 2005.

**Figure 5.5    Coverage of Safe Water and Improved Sanitation (Latrine) Services in Rural Afghanistan as Provided by the National Solidarity Program, 2005**

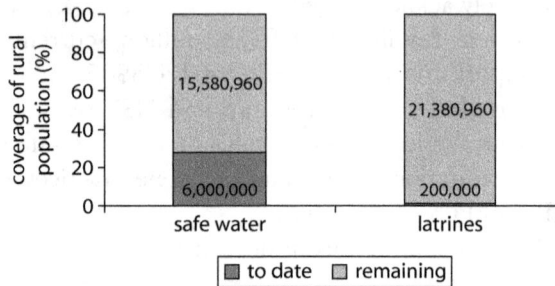

*Source:* NSS 2007.

The MRRD's NSP faces the following challenges:

- The structure of the NSP allows communities to determine for themselves their specific needs, which increases the sense of ownership for interventions but prevents everyone from receiving the complete package of water, hygiene, and sanitation services. Resources given to the NSP have a high likelihood of being spent on improved water sources but cannot be earmarked for such use.
- The NSP CDCs offer a nationwide mechanism for reaching rural areas with promotional messages (for example, nutrition or the National Hand Washing with Soap Campaign). The *Lancet* series found that counseling on hand washing can lead to a 30 percent reduction in childhood diarrhea (Bhutta and others 2008).
- The NSP faces a budget shortfall. For 2008, the budget required to scale up NSP activities to meet community-desired goals was US$65 million. Funds allocated totaled US$16.5 million, resulting in a shortfall of US$48.5 million.

### Care for Women and Children
Most interventions pertaining to care for women and children have been discussed under Pillar 3, direct nutrition interventions. Those interventions not yet discussed are included here.

***Birth spacing.*** According to the NRVA 2007/08, contraception use is low, at 15 percent overall, with 13 percent use in rural areas and 28 percent in urban areas (CSO 2009). However, coverage has increased from 5.1 percent in 2003 (UNICEF 2003). The NRVA 2007/08 also found that women with at least a primary education were twice as likely to use modern contraceptives as those with no formal education (31 percent versus 14 percent). Options available to couples include condoms, contraceptive pills, injections, intrauterine devices, and sterilization. Closely spaced pregnancies can lead to anemia and deficiencies in multiple nutrients. Birth spacing is therefore critical to protect women's health, health of newborns, and overall well-being of Afghan families. The MOPH, through its prenatal care services, Reproductive Health Department, and related adolescent health programs, strives to increase awareness and use of contraception. The nutritional study in Balkh province included men's focus groups where this issue was raised. Anemia (*kamkhuni*, or "little blood") was a highly salient issue, and men responded positively to the idea that women could have children every two or three years instead of every year. They noted that frequent pregnancies led to weaker women, weaker children, and a strain on family resources (Levitt, Pelletier, and Pell 2009). Approaching the issue as birth spacing rather than birth control (or termination) was deemed locally acceptable.

Reproductive health services offer several opportunities:

- Inadequate use of birth spacing services contributes to increased risk of maternal and child undernutrition (and death). BPHS health facilities are able to provide these services.
- Greater use of family planning services should be promoted through culturally appropriate channels.
- The media also serve as a useful mechanism for disseminating promotional messages. In the study in Balkh province, men were more likely to listen to the radio whereas women watched television.

**Women's mental health.**  Poor maternal mental health is associated with inadequate infant feeding practices. Before the BPHS took over the TFUs, the French NGO Action Contre la Faim included maternal psychosocial support as a component of its treatment package. The revised BPHS includes support for a mental health department to oversee a range of mental health services, although this work has not yet been funded. At the provincial and district hospital levels, a health worker (typically a doctor) is to serve as the mental health focal point. This person receives additional training in mental health care. In addition to seeing patients, the focal point supervises trained mental health workers at the comprehensive and basic health center levels.

The BPHS stipulates that mental health training will be provided to staff members at every level of the health system, including the community level. A psychosocial counselor or supervisor is to work in close association with the hospital-based focal point. The psychosocial counselors or supervisors are midlevel health workers (for example, nurses) with training in psychosocial counseling, according to the approved and standardized training manuals of the MOPH Mental Health Department. These counselors will have knowledge and skills necessary to provide psychosocial interventions and counseling to patients with mental disorders and patients who suffer from mental distress but do not have a formal disorder. Counselors are to work closely with the doctors and are part of the referral system within the BPHS. Their duties include supervising the basic psychosocial interventions to be implemented by the staff of the basic health centers and health posts (CHWs).

Treatment options are available in low-income contexts (Patel and others 2007).[5] A recent review reveals that the recommended time to identify women with postpartum depression is in the weeks after childbirth. In this review, Kerac and others (2010, 171–72) write:

> Among the tools specifically developed for the detection of post-natal depression, the EPDS (Edinburgh Post-Natal Depression Scale) is the most widely used in the research. It is a self-report scale of 10 questions. Each item is coded from 0 to 3 with a total ranging 0 to 30. A threshold of 12/13 suggests major depressive symptomatology but it is recommended that all women with a score of 9/10 are considered for an in-depth clinical interview. EPDS scores do not constitute diagnosis but rapid identification of potential cases. The scale has been translated and adapted in numerous contexts; the thresholds vary depending on the country. Its use is relatively easy, interview time is short, and it is well accepted by the women.

> . . .

> Effective treatments exist and may even be integrated into the routine services. In a recent study, Rahman [and others 2008] compared the impact of a cognitive-behavioral approach versus routine follow-up by the primary health agents in the rural communities of Pakistan. At six months, 23 percent of the women of the intervention group and 53 percent of the women of the control group still had a diagnosis of major depression (significant difference between the intervention group and the control group). These effects would endure at 12 months. This study illustrated the feasibility of integrating treatment for [maternal] depression with primary health services.

> . . .

Since depression constitutes a risk factor of infant malnutrition, we can make the assumption that the treatment of maternal depression will decrease the risk of infant malnutrition.

In the Afghan context, even if strategies are available, the challenge is providing the necessary training to front-line health care workers who will be able to identify and intervene in a timely manner. CHWs, midwives, vaccinators, nurses, and doctors are some of the health system personnel who would interact with pregnant and postpartum women. The family health action groups forming in some communities would be another mechanism for providing support groups. With 66 percent of the adult population estimated as depressed, services are critical.

The following gaps remain with respect to care practices for women and children:

- Culturally sensitive strategies are needed to improve use of birth spacing interventions.
- Increased funding is needed for scaling up mental health support services in general, but particularly for women during reproductive years.
- It would be beneficial to link services to the TFU facility as well.

*Social protection programs supporting care for women and children.* The Ministry of Labor, Social Affairs, Martyrs, and Disabled (MOLSAMD) supports a variety of social protection programs relevant to nutrition, covering nearly 2.5 million people. The interventions cover several groups: (a) martyrs' families—225,000, (b) people with war-related disabilities—88,000, (c) orphans and children enrolled in kindergartens (discussed later), (d) victims of natural disasters, (e) pensioners—54,000, and (f) the unemployed. Interventions include the National Skills Development Program, which assists various categories of vulnerable households; cash transfers for martyrs' families and people with disabilities; and other social services (for example, pension programs, kindergartens, and orphanages). Thirty-five percent of National Skills Development Program beneficiaries are required to be women from chronically poor, female-headed households with small children.

With support from the World Bank, a new pilot social protection program is being developed to assist vulnerable households with large numbers of children. Conditional cash transfers are being considered as a strategic approach. Two thousand families will participate during June to

October 2010 across two provinces (to be determined). The MRRD's CDCs will assist in selecting vulnerable households.

The MOLSAMD supports 32 orphanages providing care to approximately 10,500 children. The orphanages will expand services to include day-care centers so as to serve a much larger number of vulnerable children. Children receive food, hygiene instruction, literacy training, regular medical checkups, and reintegration into the education system. Nutrition promotion could be added to the existing curriculum. Assisting children with repatriation into families is another objective of the program, because about two-thirds of children in the orphanages have at least one living parent but may have been brought to the facility because of the family's poor economic status. Under the MOLSAMD's leadership and through NGOs, parents will be supported in bringing their children home. Willing families will be provided with employment opportunities, training in skills development, and grants to begin their own small businesses. Nutrition promotion could be integrated into this support package.

Kindergartens represent an easy opportunity for nutrition intervention, although participating children (estimated at 25,000) are typically from government workers' households and therefore not the most vulnerable. Opportunities exist to influence the curriculum.

The following gaps and opportunities remain with respect to these programs:

- Nutrition promotion modules were welcomed in the training programs for the National Skills Development Program, pilot social protection programs, orphanages, and kindergartens (the MOLSAMD partnered with the MOPH's PND and the MAIL's HED). The Social Protection Sector Strategy highlights the importance of reducing child undernutrition as one of the benchmarks of the Afghanistan Compact, which suggests high-level political support for nutrition in the MOLSAMD.
- Food-for-work, food-for-training, food-for-education, or simple direct food aid (for example, to vulnerable provinces such as Daykundi) distribution programs may be pursued in collaboration with the MOLSAMD, which is constructing 12 regional storage facilities for aid distribution.
- For older children (especially girls), orphanages should be linked with the HED's trainings on food security and nutrition promotion to reach girls with critical health and nutrition information before they become mothers (see accompanying photo).

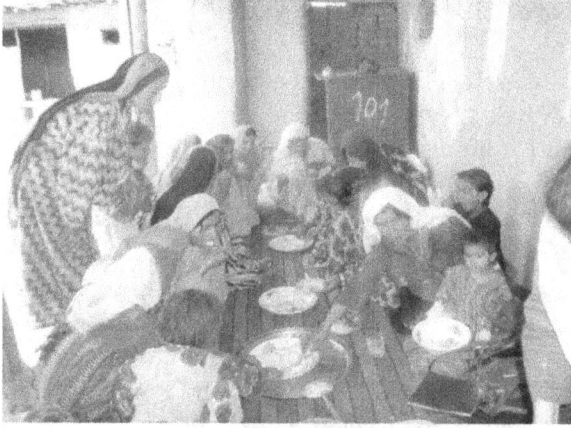

The MAIL's HED officers train vulnerable women in improved feeding practices for young children through various community platforms. Photo courtesy of FAO-Afghanistan.

## Nutrition Promotion to the General Public

Research into causes of undernutrition in Afghanistan among policy makers and implementers found that the population's lack of nutrition knowledge is a key constraint to both individual and institutional progress toward improved population nutrition (Levitt, Pelletier, and Pell 2009). Little basic nutrition information has been provided to the Afghan general public (compared to universal salt iodization or breastfeeding promotion). Schools do not routinely provide this information to students, nor do universities have training programs on the subject. There is no commonly used food guide promoting a balanced diet.

The MOPH's Preventive Health Directorate has a strong interest in nutrition promotion (particularly regarding nutrition and disease). The directorate believes the population urgently needs information on both undernutrition and problems related to nutrition and chronic disease. Fats and oils using trans fats have invaded the Afghan marketplace. Some MOPH authorities are very concerned about the transition from consumption of domestic natural oils (such as flaxseed oil) to unhealthy oils, which they believe is linked to the increasing prevalence of cardiovascular disease and premature heart attacks in the population. This health transition was also reportedly observed in northern Pakistan when foreign foods replaced local foods in the diet. Local foods had become world famous as components of a diet that supported extreme longevity (100–120 years of age).

A number of interventions have been initiated to address this information gap. However, they all remain relatively small in scale—because of limited support from development partners rather than a lack of a scalable model (most are TOT models). Another constraint is limited staff capacity within health facilities (which lost their health promotion officer in facilities during the creation of the BPHS). Formerly, nutrition guidance posters were hung on the walls of some clinics, but general nutrition promotion on a balanced diet (for example, different food groups) is not a part of the current BPHS framework.

During 2003 to 2007, colleagues from the health and agriculture sectors worked together to develop a wide range of nutrition education materials (box 5.9). These materials are used to promote nutrition through the media (radio and television), health facilities, literacy classes, schools (in particular through the MAIL and Ministry of Education), and agricultural projects.

From 2003 to 2005, the MOPH PND worked with various partners to produce a booklet, poster, and training module on basic nutrition and a more extensive training program concept note for soliciting future support from development partners. Training sessions were held on public nutrition topics for Afghan policy makers and program-level stakeholders (for example, MOPH and MAIL officers, midwives, CHWs, agriculture extension workers, local NGOs, and university professors), with the

---

**Box 5.9**

### Behavior Change Communication Activities since 2002

- Development of nutrition education materials: "Nutrition Education for Afghan Families" booklet and poster (MOPH and Tufts, reprinted with FAO); "Afghan Family Nutrition Guide" (MAIL and MOPH with FAO support)
- Integration of nutrition education in the media (radio), in health facilities, and in a broad range of community development projects (FAO)
- Integration of nutrition and food security messages in literacy materials (FAO, UN Habitat, UNICEF, WHO)
- Integration of nutrition education messages in schools (FAO, MAIL, UNICEF, WHO)

intention that information then would be passed to the community level through these conduits. These training programs have not been evaluated to determine changes in knowledge, attitudes, and practices.

Subsequent to 2005, the MOPH and MAIL jointly published in English, Dari, and Pashto nutrition reference materials. These materials included a nutrition education booklet and companion poster, the "Afghan Family Nutrition Guide" (adapted from the FAO Family Nutrition Guide) and "Healthy Food, Happy Baby, Lively Family: Improved Feeding Practices and Recipes for Afghan Children and Mothers." FAO reported that nearly 30,000 households have participated in trainings across four provinces using these nutrition education materials (FAO 2007). Locally recommended strategies for raising awareness are shown in table 5.3.

Gaps and opportunities for promoting nutrition to the general public:

- Although various tools have been developed, interventions implemented to date have occurred in only five provinces because of limited funding available through FAO (not the lack of available trained staff members to conduct these trainings). FAO reports that nearly 30,000 households have participated in these training programs as of late 2008, which represents a small proportion of the Afghan population.
- Behavior change requires proper counseling, adaptation of messages to caregivers' circumstances, transfer of skills, and peer support. Whether all these conditions are met in the current program is not

**Table 5.3    Locally Recommended Strategies for Raising Nutrition Awareness**

| Audience strategy | Men | Women | Children |
|---|---|---|---|
| Women trainers | | X | X |
| House visits | | X | X |
| Teaching at mosque | X | | |
| Farmer trainings | X | | |
| Government schools | | X (invite mothers) | X |
| Religious schools | | | X |
| Clinic workers teach at clinics or in villages | X | X | X |
| CHWs | X | X | X |
| Education of elders | X | X | |
| Radio | X | X | X |
| Television | X | X | X |
| Printed materials (books, pamphlets) | X | X | X |
| Shopkeepers (nutrition-related products such as iodized salt, oral rehydration solution, soap) | X | X | X |

*Source:* Emily Levitt (unpublished data from 2007).

clear; thus behavior change may be limited. Evaluation of the effectiveness of different basic nutrition guidance strategies to the public would be a valuable contribution.

## Pillar 5: Coordinated Support for Nutrition Is Provided by Development Partners

Within the MOPH, development partners (for example, the Asian Development Bank, the Canadian International Development Agency, the European Commission, the Japan International Cooperation Agency, the U.K. Department for International Development, USAID, and the World Bank) participate in the Consultative Group for Health and Nutrition with higher-level ministry officials. The consultative group has a broader meeting to address general policy concerns as well as a technical advisory group. The degree to which nutrition is discussed in the Consultative Group for Health and Nutrition depends on the level of involvement of the MOPH's PND, the MAIL's HED, and their international nutrition counterparts (for example, FAO, MI, UNICEF, and the WHO). Nutrition is discussed more in the technical advisory group.

As noted under Pillar 1, neither development partners nor higher-level ministry officials in either the health or agriculture sectors perceive nutrition as a high priority. However, individual interviews with these stakeholders revealed that they were not opposed to nutrition (in fact, they recognized it as essential to human survival); rather, their technical understanding of nutrition issues and the significance of nutrition for improved health and productivity was limited and thus contributed to low issue salience. One study of policy makers in Afghanistan (expatriate and Afghan) showed that neither health nor agriculture sector professionals received adequate training in topics related to human undernutrition that could inform policy decisions (Levitt, Pelletier, and Pell 2009). To increase salience of nutrition, a coalition of nutrition advocates will need to approach the respective ministers to explain the importance of nutrition and of donor commitment available to support it.

Support for research, advocacy, and communication is not coordinated in a consistent manner but rather operates project to project. Existing coordination mechanisms specific to nutrition occur largely through the Nutrition Task Force (coordinated by the MOPH's PND) and the UN system.

### Nutrition Task Force

The MOPH's PND has continued to assemble its partners on an as-needed basis for policy and programmatic discussions. This task force consists of the MAIL and other relevant ministries (varying by technical issue), FAO, MI, UNICEF, the WHO, the WFP, and NGOs. The original thematic task forces are also reassembled as needed (for example, the IYCF Task Force and Community-Based Food Security Task Force). The MOPH has also established a task force on Community-Based Management of Acute Malnutrition (with WFP and UNICEF support).

### The UN-Organized Task Forces

A renewed interest in agriculture and food security has arisen partly in reaction to the food crisis of 2008. The High-Level Task Force on the Global Food Crisis (comprising FAO, the United Nations Assistance Mission in Afghanistan, UNICEF, the WFP, the WHO, and the World Bank) under the leadership of the resident coordinator agreed to support the establishment of an Agriculture Task Force jointly led by the resident coordinator and the government of Afghanistan. This task force examines the need for emergency food aid across the country and related programs. The UN agencies recognize that the response must tackle a host of issues (for example, agriculture, health, irrigation, and social affairs) and should thus involve all development partners.

The Agriculture Task Force deals primarily with medium- and long-term programs. Established in April 2008, a Food Security Cluster (co-chaired by FAO and the WFP) and Nutrition Cluster (co-chaired by UNICEF and FAO) have been facilitating integrated and more effective action for the emergency response. The MAIL is now actively developing its implementation and coordination capacity to oversee agricultural development programs, food security surveillance, and emergency response.

Nutrition coordination efforts have improved since the establishment of the Nutrition Cluster, which was the first pilot cluster globally and led to innovations in the emergency appeal, such as the inclusion of multiple micronutrient powders. The cluster focuses on emergency interventions and community-based management of acute malnutrition as implemented through BPHS NGOs. Because food security is addressed through a separate cluster, the integration of health and food security interventions remains limited.

## The Joint Program

A Joint Program on Children, Food Security, and Nutrition in Afghanistan has been initiated by agriculture and health sector stakeholders. In 2009, partial funding was received from the Spanish Millennium Development Goals Trust Fund. Activities are set to commence in early 2010. The goal of the program is to contribute to the reduction of undernutrition through sustainable and multisectoral efforts at community, district, provincial, and central levels and to contribute to the achievement of the Millennium Development Goals in Afghanistan. The program's strategy is structured around two outcomes, both designed to integrate a broad range of expertise and activities addressing the symptoms and the immediate and underlying causes of undernutrition:

- *Outcome 1* focuses on the implementation of a comprehensive package of *community-level* nutrition and food security interventions and thus contributes directly to the reduction of undernutrition at the district level.
- *Outcome 2* focuses on strengthening the *policy frameworks and institutional mechanisms* required to support integrated nutrition interventions (including nutrition advocacy, mainstreaming, and information management and coordination) and thus contributes to a reduction of undernutrition in the longer term. Outcome 2 lays the foundations for nutrition and food security activities to be scaled up and sustained beyond the end of the program.

The package includes nutrition education, IYCF and family nutrition counseling (including breastfeeding counseling and training in the preparation of improved complementary foods), community-based management of acute malnutrition, improving nutrition services provided through health facilities, household food production and income-generation activities, and nutrition monitoring and impact assessment in project areas. The package will have very limited coverage initially: it will be implemented in only 10 food insecure and underserved districts of Afghanistan (in up to five provinces).

## Notes

1. Personal communication, Laird Ruth, International Micronutrient Malnutrition Prevention and Control program, U.S. Centers for Disease Control and Prevention, Atlanta, October 2009.

2. Personal communication, Ibrahim Parvanta, independent consultant, former director of International Micronutrient Malnutrition Prevention and Control program, U.S. Centers for Disease Control and Prevention, Atlanta, October 2009.

3. The focus group was held during an in-service training of PNOs, July 23, 2009, in Kabul.

4. Personal communication, MRRD Deputy Minister Ahmad Barmak and Senior Adviser Hermione Youngs, Kabul, July 2009.

5. The Center for Justice and Peacebuilding at Eastern Mennonite University (Harrisonburg, Virginia) works in numerous postconflict zones using the STAR (Strategies for Trauma Awareness and Resilience) trauma recovery program. More information can be found at http://www.emu.edu/cjp/star/trauma-healing-seminars. Among the economies that have participated in the STAR program are Burundi, Colombia, Croatia, Mexico, Sudan, and the West Bank and Gaza.

## References

Berti, Peter R., Julia Krasevec, and Sian FitzGerald. 2004. "A Review of the Effectiveness of Agriculture Interventions in Improving Nutrition Outcomes." *Public Health Nutrition* 7 (5): 599–609.

Bhutta, Zulfiqar A., Tahmeed Ahmed, Robert E. Black, Simon Cousens, Kathryn Dewey, Elsa Giugliani, Batool A. Haider, Betty Kirkwood, Saul S. Morris, H. P. S. Sachdev, and Meera Shekar. 2008. "What Works? Interventions for Maternal and Child Undernutrition and Survival." *Lancet* 371 (9608): 417–40.

Brun, Thierry, Jacqueline Reynaud, and Simon Chevassus-Agnes. 1989. "Food and Nutritional Impact of One Home Garden Project in Senegal." *Ecology of Food and Nutrition* 23 (2): 91–108.

CSO (Central Statistics Office). 2009. *National Risk and Vulnerability Assessment 2007/08: A Profile of Afghanistan*. Kabul: Ministry of Rural Rehabilitation and Development.

English, Ruth, and Jacqui Badcock. 1998. "A Community Nutrition Project in Viet Nam: Effects on Child Morbidity." *Food, Nutrition, and Agriculture* 22: 15–22.

FAO (Food and Agriculture Organization). 2007. "Supporting Household Food Security, Nutrition and Livelihoods in Afghanistan, GCP/AFG/039/GER: Project Findings and Recommendations." FAO, Kabul.

Griffiths, Marcia, Kate Dickin, and Michael Favin. 1996. "Promoting the Growth of Children: What Works." Human Development Department, World Bank, Washington, DC.

Kennedy, Eileen T., and Harold Alderman. 1987. *Comparative Analyses of Nutritional Effectiveness of Food Subsidies and Other Food-Related Interventions.* Washington, DC: International Food Policy Research Institute.

Kerac, Marko, Marie McGrath, Carlos Grijalva-Eternod, Cecile Bizouerne, Jenny Saxton, Heather Bailey, Caroline Wilkinson, June Hirsch, Hannah Blencowe, Jeremy Shoham, and Andrew Seal. 2010. *Management of Acute Malnutrition in Infants (MAMI) Project: Technical Review—Current Evidence, Policies, Practices, and Programme Outcomes.* London: Emergency Nutrition Network. http://www.ennonline.net/pool/files/ife/mami-report-complete%281%29.pdf.

Levitt, Emily. 2005. "Growth Monitoring and Promotion in Afghanistan: A Review of Policy and Practice." Ministry of Public Health, Kabul.

Levitt, Emily J., David L. Pelletier, and Alice N. Pell. 2009. "Revisiting the UNICEF Malnutrition Framework to Foster Agriculture and Health Sector Collaboration to Reduce Malnutrition: A Comparison of Stakeholder Priorities for Action." *Food Policy* 34 (2): 156–65.

Levitt, Emily J., Rebecca J. Stoltzfus, David L. Pelletier, and Alice N. Pell. 2009. "A Community Food System Analysis as Formative Research for a Comprehensive Anemia Control Program in Northern Afghanistan." *Food Security* 1 (2): 177–95.

Marsh, Robin. 1998. "Building on Traditional Gardening to Improve Household Food Security." *Food, Nutrition, and Agriculture* 22 (5): 4–13.

MOPH (Ministry of Public Health). 2006. *Afghanistan Health Survey 2006: Estimates of Priority Health Indicators for Rural Afghanistan.* Kabul: MOPH.

———. 2009. "Strategy on Prevention and Control of Vitamin and Mineral Deficiencies in Afghanistan." Public Nutrition Department, MOPH, Kabul.

MOPH (Ministry of Public Health), UNICEF (United Nations Children's Fund), CDC (Centers for Disease Control and Prevention), National Institute for Research on Food and Nutrition–Italy, and Tufts University. 2009. *2004 Afghanistan National Nutrition Survey.* Atlanta: CDC.

NSS (National Surveillance System). 2007. *The National Risk and Vulnerability Assessment 2005: Afghanistan.* Kabul: Ministry of Rural Rehabilitation and Development and the Central Statistics Office.

Patel, Vikram, Ricardo Araya, Sudipto Chatterjee, Dan Chisholm, Alex Cohen, Mary De Silva, Clemens Hosman, Hugh McGuire, Graciela Rojas, and Mark van Ommeren. 2007. "Treatment and Prevention of Mental Disorders in Low-Income and Middle-Income Countries." *Lancet* 370 (9591): 991–1005.

Rahman, Atif, Abid Malik, Siham Sikander, Christopher Roberts, and Francis Creed. 2008. "Cognitive Behaviour Therapy-Based Intervention by Community Health Workers for Mothers with Depression and Their Infants in Rural Pakistan: A Cluster-Randomised Controlled Trial." *Lancet* 372 (9642): 902–9.

Reji, Gedlu S. 2007. "Final Report on MRRD-UNCHR WATSAN Program Evaluation." Ministry of Rural Rehabilitation and Development and United Nations High Commissioner for Refugees, Kabul.

UNICEF (United Children's Fund). 2003. *Multiple Indicator Cluster Survey.* Kabul: UNICEF.

CHAPTER 6

# Recommendations

Recommendations for policy and programmatic action are presented corresponding to the nutrition investment framework, which developed out of the Global Action Plan for Nutrition.

## Pillar 1: Nutrition Is Recognized as Foundational to National Development

This section outlines the needs related to policy-level support for nutrition and new institutional arrangements for creating or sustaining support for nutrition in Afghanistan.

Nutrition is not currently recognized as a strategic investment for national development. There is no overarching national nutrition action plan with targets and cost estimates. At high levels, nutrition is currently viewed as a subcomponent of other sectoral policies. The health and agriculture sectors have nutrition plans, and other sectoral plans contain nutrition-related aspects, but the ministries are limited in their ability to coordinate multisectoral nutrition activities.

Advocacy is required to make the case for nutrition as a strategic national investment in the health and agriculture sectors as well as in the education sector, among others. Specifically, nutrition-related departments are inadequately placed and supported in government organizational, operational, and funding structures. Conducting a PROFILES[1] exercise to demonstrate the effect of undernutrition on the country's development would further support advocacy efforts.

The Afghanistan National Development Strategy contains a precedent to create a nutrition cross-cutting strategy on the basis of its six other cross-cutting strategies (see appendix F). This approach would involve creation of a high-level committee for nutrition (for example, a consultative group) to oversee a multisectoral strategy and costed action plan. The committee would plan multisectorally, and each sector would implement its agreed-on programs. This approach has been adopted for the Gender Equity Cross-Cutting Strategy. National cross-sectoral goals are set, but the line ministries implement them within their areas of responsibility and are then held accountable under the national gender agenda.

Independent of the creation of a new institutional structure and coordination mechanism, greater support is needed for existing government departments working in nutrition, such as the Public Nutrition Department (PND) of the Ministry of Public Health (MOPH) and Home Economics Department (HED) of the Ministry of Agriculture, Irrigation, and Livestock (MAIL).

## Pillar 2: Adequate Local Capacity Is Built and Supported to Design and Execute Effective Nutrition Policies and Programs

Sustaining support for nutrition at the highest levels will require a greater investment in building local capacity. Government health and agriculture sector staff members have in-service and short-course training in nutrition but no formal degree training. Support is needed for some government staff members to receive either distance-learning training or training abroad at least at the master's degree level in nutritional science, supplemented with training in policy development and program management.

The absence of undergraduate or graduate-level degree programs in nutrition in Afghanistan means support is needed for the development of nutrition training programs through local institutions. Some encouraging initiatives are currently under way and could be expanded. The U.S. Agency for International Development (USAID) has funded the University of Massachusetts Amherst to support a curriculum revision at Kabul Medical University. The University of Massachusetts is planning to include a nutrition course in its undergraduate curriculum, and two or three nutrition courses in a new master's of public health program set for

2010. Also, the joint program funded by the Spanish Millennium Development Goals Trust Fund includes support for nutrition training through the Health Sciences Institute (for nurses and midwives). Cheragh Medical Institute, a private institution in Kabul seeking university status, has expressed interest in providing nutrition training, but it currently has no partners to actualize this goal.

A major constraint in executing policies remains inadequate control over resources for nutrition. Neither the PND nor the HED has an adequate core operating budget; both have to request funds for each activity through their development partners. An improved procurement mechanism or more streamlined process would greatly facilitate nutrition program delivery and potentially win support from development partners for nutrition.

The operational needs of key ministries also should be addressed. Additional operational capacity needs of the PND include improved transportation for coordination with partners and monitoring (for example, a budget for car rental); communications for supervision of provincial staff members and partners (for example, Internet, phone); and culturally appropriate meeting spaces for women to attend events (for example, government-owned spaces rather than hotels).

The weakness in community outreach for behavior change to improve nutrition also needs to be addressed. It will be important to draw lessons from the approach currently being implemented by USAID's Basic Support for Institutionalizing Child Survival (BASICS) Project and to scale up successful elements of that approach. Putting in place a system of female community nutrition workers, similar to successful models currently operating at scale in Nepal and Pakistan, could be considered.

## Pillar 3: Cost-Effective, Direct Nutrition Interventions are Scaled Up, Where Applicable

The following recommendations could be achieved through the MOPH's Basic Package of Health Services (BPHS):

- Support the BPHS and the Essential Package of Hospital Services in ensuring that staff members are providing correct nutrition messages. A seven-module training is available from the PND and can be taught in Kabul as well as in the provinces by provincial nutrition officers. As previously noted, additional community nutrition workers may need to be hired to implement the nutrition components of the BPHS.

- Increase awareness in the health sector and general public about the importance of iron and folic acid early in pregnancy (for example, by conducting a media campaign, by instituting a Ministry of Women's Affairs and MOPH–supported annual Women's Health Week, or by partnering with the MAIL to reach girls through the schools or with the Ministry of Youth Affairs to reach girls before they are engaged).
- In parallel with expansion of prenatal care coverage, consider including multiple micronutrient supplements and food supplements for under-weight mothers as part of a conditional prenatal care program. Food supplements can reduce the number of infants born small for their gestational age by 32 percent among mothers with low body mass index (Bhutta and others 2008). Pilot-testing is critical because women may be underweight during pregnancy by choice, out of fear of having a baby too large to deliver. Some women undereat in the latter trimesters because of concern about obstructed labor. Messages that address these concerns and improved access to emergency obstetric care would allay some fears.
- Scale up breastfeeding counselor trainings through the MOPH's PND national and provincial staff and consider including this intervention in performance-based financing schemes to all mothers during prena-tal care and those who deliver in a BPHS facility. Exit interviews with patients can be used for verification. Consider certifying all trained midwives also as breastfeeding counselors because they have immediate access to women during pregnancy and the early postpartum period. Quality control will be important to ensure that proper messages are being provided to mothers.
- Improve coverage of postpartum vitamin A by stimulating demand through the BPHS, media, and related community channels (for example, community health workers, family health action groups, and an annual Women's Health Week campaign).
- Improve coverage (demand and use) of deworming treatments for pregnant women and preschool children.
- Collaborate with the MOPH's PND, the Micronutrient Initiative, and the United Nations Children's Fund (UNICEF) to explore an alternative delivery mechanism for child vitamin A supplementation beyond the National Immunization Days (for example, a Child Health Week).
- Improve community-level programming through mechanisms such as support groups (for example, family health action groups) for infant and young child feeding; diarrhea management (with oral rehydration solution and zinc); deworming; referrals for the Expanded Programme

on Immunization and treatment of infections; and maternal health care. Coordinate with USAID's BASICS III Project to learn of the effect of its pilot growth promotion program as a platform for maternal and child health and nutrition programming.[2]

- Ensure that adequate funding is provided for scaling up zinc supplementation with oral rehydration solution for diarrhea treatment.
- Continue hygiene promotion through BPHS facilities and community support structures.
- Continue support of therapeutic feeding units, and investigate why wasting is so high in children one to two years of age.
- Expand geographic coverage of the Community-Based Management of Acute Malnutrition program to treat not only especially severely malnourished children but also moderately malnourished children to prevent them from becoming severely malnourished.
- Develop business models for the introduction of low-cost fortified complementary foods and micronutrient powders, such as Sprinkles, through commercial channels.

The following nutrition promotion efforts could be accomplished through agriculture and broader sectoral partnerships:

- With the MOPH's PND and MAIL's HED, develop a program for general promotion of nutrition, which could include developing a basic nutrition education diagram (for example, a food group pyramid); supporting reproduction of nutrition promotion materials (in Dari and Pashto as well as versions for illiterate audiences); and using various media to fill the gap in public awareness about the basics of a balanced diet.

- Scale up complementary feeding (and broad infant and young child feeding) promotion activities through multiple community-level platforms (for example, the MAIL's Horticulture and Livestock Project producer groups; HED's women's self-help groups; the Ministry of Rural Rehabilitation and Development's National Solidarity Program women's community development committees; the Ministry of Women's Affairs women's literacy circles; the Ministry of Labor, Social Affairs, Martyrs, and Disabled's orphanages and kindergartens). Include innovations such as multiple micronutrient powders and an evaluation component to determine the most effective strategies (and packaged approaches) to achieve behavior change in complementary feeding practices.

- Combine nutrition promotion activities with activities to improve household food security in food-insecure areas. These activities may include conditional cash transfers, support for food processing, preservation, and storage income-generating trainings, or microcredit support for other income-generating activities (for example, Horticulture and Livestock Project programs). Include an evaluation component to assess program strengths and areas for improvement.

- Scale up the school-based nutrition education program to reach boys and girls because this training reaches them before they become engaged and start families. It is when girls are most accessible. Include a component on nutrition through the life course for girls and, if possible, boys because the latter will be future providers and do most of the food purchasing. Girls and boys attend school at different times, so this approach would be feasible. Include an evaluation component to assess changes in knowledge, attitudes, and practices.

The following could be accomplished through public-private partnerships:

- Work with partners to address the critical bottleneck of contaminated domestic salt supply through a salt purification facility. Coordinate with the MOPH, the Micronutrient Initiative, and UNICEF.
- Subsequent to improvements in quality of domestic salt, conduct a media campaign to regain consumer confidence in domestic salt.
- Pursue double fortification of salt with both iron and iodine because small-scale flour fortification has proved impractical in the current context and large-scale flour millers currently reach less than 10 percent of the population.
- Support formation of a flour millers' association in Afghanistan to work with the existing salt producers' association on coordination, quality control, and mutual accountability.
- Support legislation on flour fortification using new World Health Organization standards (iron, folate, zinc, vitamin $B_{12}$, and vitamin A) and a mechanism such as the Afghanistan National Standards Authority for enforcement.
- Conduct a market feasibility study of multiple micronutrient powders for home-based fortification for children (for example, Sprinkles,

Anuka). Use of these powders can reduce anemia risk in children by 21 percent (Bhutta and others 2008).

- Explore a public-private partnership for extending the reach of Nutrition Zenda, the fortified complementary food currently produced by a small business in Kabul. Support for similar products should also be explored.
- Engage with the Horticulture and Livestock Project's dairy program about fortifying milk with vitamins A and D. Initial investigation of this possibility was met with interest from the project's technical advisers. This effort may reach only selected urban areas (large cities), but the private sector may assume the cost of the fortificant so it represents a low-hanging-fruit opportunity. Explore oil and ghee fortification with vitamin A. This effort may be pursued through coordination with importers or directly with local producers.

## Pillar 4: Determinants of Undernutrition Are Addressed through Multisectoral Approaches

This multisectoral approach specifically implies multisectoral collaboration for high-level planning purposes and then sectoral implementation of policies and programs appropriate to each sector. The sectors then convene at agreed-on intervals to assess progress toward shared national nutrition goals.

The following goals can be achieved through the Ministry of Agriculture, Irrigation, and Livestock:

- Provide support to strengthen and coordinate routine food security surveillance (early-warning system) activities in the country.
- Evaluate the HED's training-of-trainer activities, focusing on improving household food security and women's income generation, to determine whether these activities should be scaled up as is or reformed. Opportunities exist to scale up in 12 additional provinces and to cover more districts in the 5 provinces with current activities.
- Continue supporting the Horticulture and Livestock Project—specifically the horticulture, dairy, and poultry programs that include men's and women's producer groups and are available platforms for nutrition promotion. Consider making support contingent on including nutrition outcomes in project evaluation (for example, changes in household consumption patterns and nutritional status).

These objectives can be met through the Ministry of Rural Rehabilitation and Development:

- Advocate for the National Risk and Vulnerability Assessment (NRVA) to continue including household food security questions (on calories and diet diversity) in the survey conducted every two years. Advocate for inclusion of vitamin A supplementation, use of iodized salt, iron and folic acid use during prenatal care, and other simple nutrition-related indicators. Explore the feasibility of including a more intensive nutritional assessment as a substudy of every other NRVA (every four years) with anthropometric data on individuals (women, children under age five, and possibly school-age children, and men). Certain other nutritional indicators could be included (for example, anemia status and use of iodized salt).
- Support the Rural Water, Sanitation, and Irrigation Program to meet the high demand for safe drinking water, improved sanitation, and hygiene promotion activities.
- Continue to support the National Solidarity Program because the top request from communities continues to be for safe drinking water. Nutrition-tagged funding could be provided through the Rural Water, Sanitation, and Irrigation Program for National Solidarity Program requests related to water, sanitation, and hygiene.
- Support a national campaign to promote hand washing, possibly as a public-private partnership to increase access to low-cost soap. Counseling on hand washing can lead to a 30 percent reduction in child diarrhea (Bhutta and others 2008). This campaign could also be done in tandem with a push to scale up access to clean water (for washing) with the Ministry of Rural Rehabilitation and Development, UNICEF, the MOPH, the Ministry of Education's Healthy Schools Initiative, and others working in hygiene promotion.

The following initiative could be accomplished through the Ministry of Labor, Social Affairs, Martyrs, and Disabled:

- Encourage social protection programs to vulnerable households to include nutrition promotion as a component of a broader package of interventions (for example, cash transfer, food for work, food for education, food security and income-generation trainings through the MAIL's HED).

## Pillar 5: Coordinated Support for Nutrition Is Provided by Development Partners

An improved mechanism is required to adequately coordinate the varied multisectoral activities related to nutrition. See the recommendations under Pillar 1.

More collective advocacy and communications on nutrition to high authorities are required by nutrition partners.

> "Every anguish passes except the anguish of hunger. . . . The world lives in hope."
>
> —Afghan proverbs

## Notes

1. PROFILES is a computer-based nutrition advocacy tool.
2. Meanwhile, USAID has decided to scale up this growth promotion program in all 13 of the USAID-supported provinces.

## Reference

Bhutta, Zulfiqar A., Tahmeed Ahmed, Robert E. Black, Simon Cousens, Kathryn Dewey, Elsa Giugliani, Batool A. Haider, Betty Kirkwood, Saul S. Morris, H. P. S. Sachdev, and Meera Shekar. 2008. "What Works? Interventions for Maternal and Child Undernutrition and Survival." *Lancet* 371 (9608): 417–40.

# Methodology

The methods used in the compilation of this report include the following:

- Network assessment
- Analysis of available nutritional epidemiology data
- Analysis of available knowledge, attitudes, and practices (KAP) data
- Review of the Basic Package of Health Services (BPHS) regarding nutrition
- Review of programs in nonhealth sectors that affect or could affect nutrition
- Assessment of the capacity of the Public Nutrition Department of the Ministry of Public Health (MOPH) and other nutrition-relevant institutional structures to lead and implement scaled-up, effective multisectoral nutrition interventions
- Selection of analytical approach

## Network Assessment

To identify the network of stakeholders in health and other sectors relevant to nutrition, the authors used the chain-referral sampling strategy. This method effectively identifies hidden or unknown populations and is a technique where initial (index) individuals recommend additional participants from among their acquaintances (Schensul, Schensul, and LeCompte 1999). In this case, index stakeholders were members of the MOPH's Public Nutrition Department, the United Nations Children's Fund (UNICEF)–Afghanistan's Nutrition Section, the Household Food Security, Nutrition, and Livelihoods Office of the Food and Agriculture Organization of the United Nations (FAO), and the staff of the Basic Support for Institutionalizing Child Survival (BASICS) III Project of the U.S. Agency for International Development (USAID). Perspectives from Afghans, expatriates, and both genders were solicited. Sectors of particular interest included health, agriculture, education, rural development, and the private sector. The objective of the chain-referral sampling strategy was to reach the informational saturation point of "sufficient redundancy"—when patterns of response repeated, generating no new relevant information (Trotter and Schensul 1998).

Initial contact was made with index stakeholders by telephone or Internet during June 2009, and arrangements were made for in-person meetings during the July 9–25, 2009, mission. More than 60 meetings were held with nutrition-relevant stakeholders during the July and subsequent October missions. This number includes multiple visits with a small number of the key index stakeholders. In-depth discussions with individuals or focus groups with multiple members of the same institution occurred during the July field mission. Information was gathered about stakeholder policies, programs, and activities pertaining to nutrition. Focus groups were held with 11 representatives from six nongovernmental organizations (NGOs) implementing the BPHS, 15 provincial nutrition officers, more than 20 male and female primary school teachers from Kabul implementing the School-Based Nutrition Program, the Nutrition Cluster (chaired by UNICEF and FAO), and the Afghanistan National Development Strategy Consultative Group on Health and Nutrition. Stakeholders were asked about the location, scale (coverage), targeting, and efficacy of programs relevant to nutrition. Successes and challenges related to the implementation of programs were documented. The follow-up mission (October 12–23, 2009) involved a meeting with the Nutrition Task Force to review recommendations in this report (BASICS III; FAO; Micronutrient Initiative; Ministry of Agriculture, Irrigation, and Livestock Home Economic Department; MOPH Public Nutrition Department; UNICEF; USAID Food for Peace;

World Food Programme; World Health Organization). Additional meetings were held to clarify components of the report. The Ministry of Education was unavailable during both field missions. As a result, education sector information was solicited from organizations working with this ministry. A matrix of selected partner activities is shown in appendix K.

## Synthesis and Analysis of Available Nutritional Epidemiology Data

Data used in this report derive largely from the 2004 National Nutrition Survey. Other data were gathered through solicitation of the network of stakeholders identified. Through a desk review, a meta-analysis of the 2004 and other existing data is included for each nutrition indicator where possible. No recurrent survey includes anthropometric indicators for nutrition, but rather a series of surveys has been conducted, using differing methodologies in varying regions and with varying indicators. Where possible, data are desegregated by gender, age, socioeconomic status, and geographic location. Data are presented for levels and trends (if possible) on undernutrition of mothers and children and related underlying causes. Data for other populations (for example, men) and overnutrition among women (for example, overweight and obesity) are also shown as available. Additional data sources are referenced as available. These are shown in appendix B.

## Analysis of Available KAP Data

Data on nutrition-related knowledge, attitudes, and practices were solicited from stakeholders. The 2004 National Nutrition Survey included some nationally representative data on selected indicators (for example, awareness of iodized salt, knowledge of vitamins). Other KAP data came from small-scale or regional studies conducted by United Nations agencies (FAO, UNICEF, World Food Programme, World Health Organization); government ministries (MOPH; Ministry of Agriculture, Irrigation, and Livestock); NGOs (Save the Children); or universities (Tufts, Cornell). A meta-analysis of these data is included in this report according to the following nutrition concerns: infant and young child feeding, maternal nutrition, micronutrients, and general nutrition knowledge.

## Review of the BPHS Regarding Nutrition

During 2009, the MOPH updated the BPHS and Essential Package of Hospital Services. Nutrition components in the finalized BPHS are shown in appendix E. The adequacy of the BPHS to address nutrition concerns through health sector channels was assessed through desk review, in-depth discussions with health sector stakeholders, and focus group meetings, particularly with six of the NGOs contracted by the MOPH to implement the BPHS. The adequacy and quality of each direct nutrition intervention is described in chapter 5 of this report.

## Review of Programs in Other (Nonhealth) Sectors That Affect or Could Affect Nutrition

Much of this analysis occurred in tandem with the network assessment previously described. These sectors were selected in relation to the underlying causes of nutritional problems highlighted in the UNICEF framework and those collaborating in work or interested in collaborations related to nutrition. These sectors included food security, health environment, social protection, education, higher education, women's affairs, commerce, mines and industry, and the private sector.

## Capacity Assessment of the MOPH's Public Nutrition Department and Other Institutional Structures to Lead and Implement Scaled-Up, Effective Multisectoral Nutrition Interventions

Institutional structures available to lead and implement scaled-up, effective multisectoral nutrition interventions were identified through the discussions held in the network assessment. Likewise, the interventions that were operating or that could be considered were identified through the same process. Where institutional structures were lacking, recommendations have been made to address this gap.

A capacity assessment was conducted of the MOPH's Public Nutrition Department and the Ministry of Agriculture, Irrigation and Livestock's Home Economics Department, the two government structures most directly responsible for nutrition interventions. Capacity assessments had been done of these two departments in 2006 to 2007 by Cornell University with funding from GRM International (Levitt 2006). These assessments were updated using a methodology from the health systems literature.

This assessment uses a four-tier hierarchy of capacity-building needs: (a) structures, systems, and roles; (b) staff and facilities; (c) skills; and (d) tools. The first tier forms the base of the capacity structure, with each successive tier building on the one before it. This systemic capacity-building framework has nine elements, categorized under various tiers. These are further described in appendix J (Potter and Brough 2004).

## Analytical Approach

The interpretation of the data is structured according to five pillars identified as necessary for progress in reducing undernutrition at the country level. These pillars are derived from the Global Action Plan for Nutrition (see chapter 1), an initiative in the international development community that is designed to increase attention and support for reducing malnutrition at scale. These pillars were identified from a review of numerous country experiences, particularly successful country case studies, and current evidence-based strategies available for nutrition. The pillars are

- *Pillar 1:* Nutrition is recognized as foundational to national development (chapter 4).
- *Pillar 2:* Adequate local capacity is built and supported to design and execute effective nutrition policies and programs (chapter 4).
- *Pillar 3:* Cost-effective, direct nutrition interventions are scaled up, where applicable. (chapter 5).
- *Pillar 4:* Determinants of undernutrition are addressed through multi-sectoral approaches (chapters 3 and 5).
- *Pillar 5:* Coordinated support for nutrition is provided by development partners (including funding for advocacy, communications, and research) (chapter 5).

This report contains recommendations to address gaps identified through this pillar-based analytical framework.

## References

Levitt, Emily. 2006. "Pursuing Food System Approaches to Promote Food Security and Reduce Malnutrition in Afghanistan." GRM International, Kabul.

Potter, Christopher, and Richard Brough. 2004. "Systemic Capacity Building: A Hierarchy of Needs." *Health Policy and Planning* 19 (5): 336–54.

Schensul, Stephen, Jean J. Schensul, and Margaret D. LeCompte. 1999. "Ethnographic Sampling." In *Essential Ethnographic Methods: Observations, Interviews, and Questionnaires*, 231–69. Walnut Creek, CA: AltaMira Press.

Trotter, Robert T., and Jean J. Schensul. 1998. "Methods in Applied Anthropology." In *Handbook of Methods in Cultural Anthropology*, ed. H. Russell Bernard, 691–736. Walnut Creek, CA: AltaMira Press.

# Nutrition Data Collection in Afghanistan

| Nutrition indicators by demographic | 2004 National Nutrition Survey[a] | Other national-level data collection |
|---|---|---|
| *Children under five years of age* | | |
| Stunting (weight for height) | Yes | — |
| Underweight (weight for age) | Yes | — |
| Wasting (weight for height) | Yes | Ministry of Public Health's Health Management Information System screening at Basic Package of Health Services facilities |
| Iodine deficiency | — | — |
| Iron deficiency | Yes | — |
| Anemia | Yes | Basic Package of Health Services screening |
| Zinc deficiency | — | None |
| Vitamin A deficiency | Unsuccessful | None |
| Vitamin A supplementation | Yes | 2006 Afghanistan Health Survey; National Immunization Days reports |
| Vitamin C deficiency | — | None |
| Vitamin D deficiency | — | One regional study under way |
| Breastfeeding initiation | — | 2006 Afghanistan Health Survey |
| Exclusive breastfeeding | — | 2006 Afghanistan Health Survey |

*(continued)*

| Nutrition indicators by demographic | 2004 National Nutrition Survey[a] | Other national-level data collection |
|---|---|---|
| Timely introduction of complementary foods | — | 2006 Afghanistan Health Survey |
| Ever breastfed during 0–24 months | — | 2006 Afghanistan Health Survey |
| *School-age children* | | |
| Anthropometry (height, weight) | — | Healthy Schools Initiative reportedly considering this |
| Micronutrients (only iodine) | Yes | — |
| *Women of reproductive age* | | |
| Anthropometry (underweight) | Yes | — |
| Iodine deficiency | Yes | — |
| Iron deficiency | Yes | — |
| Anemia | Yes | — |
| Vitamin A deficiency | (night blindness) | — |
| Iron and folic acid received during prenatal care | — | 2006 Afghanistan Health Survey |
| Breastfeeding counseling in prenatal care | — | 2006 Afghanistan Health Survey |
| *Men* | | |
| Anthropometry | — | None |
| Iron deficiency | Yes | — |
| Anemia | Yes | — |
| *Elderly* | | |
| Anthropometry | — | None |
| Micronutrient deficiencies | — | None |
| *Households* | | |
| Food consumption (including calories) | — | National Risk and Vulnerability Assessment |
| Diet diversity (food frequencies) | — | National Risk and Vulnerability Assessment |
| Perceived as food insecure | — | National Risk and Vulnerability Assessment |
| *Other* | | |
| Zinc deficiency | — | None |
| Vitamin C deficiency | — | None |
| Vitamin D deficiency | — | None |

*(continued)*

| Nutrition indicators by demographic | 2004 National Nutrition Survey[a] | Other national-level data collection |
|---|---|---|
| Crop production and food supplies (market availability, prices) | — | Ministry of Agriculture, Irrigation, and Livestock's Food, Agriculture, and Animal Husbandry Information Management and Policy Monitoring System; U.S. Agency for International Development's Famine Early Warning System; World Food Programme's Vulnerability Mapping Unit |

*Source:* MOPH and others 2009.
*Note:* — = data not collected.
a. The National Nutrition Survey also included questions related to nutrition knowledge (for example, has the respondent ever heard of vitamins, use of iodized salt, and so on).

# Reference

MOPH (Ministry of Public Health), UNICEF (United Nations Children's Fund), CDC (Centers for Disease Control and Prevention), National Institute for Research on Food and Nutrition–Italy, and Tufts University, 2009. *2004 Afghanistan National Nutrition Survey.* Atlanta: CDC.

# Cultural Beliefs Relating to Infant and Young Child Feeding

The data in the tables in this appendix have been collected through focus groups discussions carried out by Food and Agriculture Organization of the United Nations and the Afghanistan Ministry of Agriculture, Irrigation, and Livestock in a sample of villages from selected districts in three provinces of Afghanistan (Badakshan, Bamyan, and Herat) in 2006. The results cannot be considered as representative of the general population's beliefs in the provinces where they occur, but they do illustrate the type and diversity of beliefs that can be present and the ways in which nutrition education messages can be tailored in response to such beliefs.

## Beliefs about Energy-Rich Foods for Infants and Young Children

Table C.1 describes beliefs held about energy-rich foods. Comments and recommendations are as follows:

- Consider methods of preparation of staple foods (bread, rice, potatoes) to improve acceptability for infants and young children and to prevent problems with digestion (and choking). For example, well-cooked, soft rice may be more acceptable than harder grains. Bread soaked in liquids such as broths or milk may be more acceptable than fresh, dry bread.

**Table C.1    Beliefs about Energy-Rich Foods for Infants and Young Children**

| Food group | Food item | Belief | Province |
|---|---|---|---|
| *Beneficial* | | | |
| Cereals | Wheat bread | Produces energy | BD |
| | Rice | With little oil, is energetic | BM |
| | Rice (*shola*) | Soft, energetic | BD, HT |
| Roots | Potatoes | Soft, energetic, good for health | BD, HT |
| Fats | Fats | Warm, soft, useful | BD, BM, HT |
| *Harmful* | | | |
| Cereals | Wheat bread | Enlarges abdomen, hard to digest | BD, BM, HT |
| | *Kolcha* | Difficult to digest | BM |
| | *Palaw* (rice) | Difficult to digest | BD, BM, HT |
| Roots | Potatoes | Cold and hard to digest, causes stomachache | BM |
| Fats | Fats | Cause diarrhea | HT |
| Sugars | Sweets | Cause diarrhea | HT |

*Source:* Focus groups in three provinces.
*Note:* BD = Badakhshan; BM = Bamyan; HT = Herat.

- With the exception of the World Food Programme's fortified biscuits, biscuits have limited nutritional value. Soft bread, which is more affordable and available, would be a suitable alternative to biscuits. Biscuits that are similar to cookies present problems for dental health if tooth brushing is not practiced.
- Moderate use of fats was acceptable to respondents and may be encouraged. Overuse is believed to cause diarrhea.
- Sweets were not valued and could be harmful in causing diarrhea. Avoid promoting sweets because more appropriate energy sources are available to local communities. Moderate use of sweeteners for foods, such as honey or sugar, may be considered because no harmful effects were noted.

## Beliefs about Protein-Rich Foods for Infants and Young Children

Beliefs about protein-rich foods are described in table C.2. Comments and recommendations follow:

- Milk, yogurt, and eggs may be promoted as proteins for infants and young children after advance pilot-testing of promotional materials locally to learn about preparation methods that would decrease certain

**Table C.2    Beliefs about Protein-Rich Foods for Infants and Young Children**

| Food group | Food item | Belief | Province |
|---|---|---|---|
| *Beneficial* | | | |
| Dairy | Milk | Energetic, useful | BD, BM, HT |
| | Yogurt | Hot, good for baby | HT |
| Eggs | Eggs | Energetic, nutritious | BM, HT |
| *Harmful* | | | |
| Dairy | Buttermilk | Cold, causes pneumonia and edema | BM |
| | Cow milk | Hard to digest, causes diarrhea | BD |
| | Yogurt | Causes stomachache | BD |
| Eggs | Eggs | Delay child's speaking | BD, BM |
| Meat | Meat | Hard to digest, makes baby sick, causes abdominal problems, causes baby to eat soil | BD, BM, HT |
| | Beef | Hard to digest | BM |
| | Broth | Causes diarrhea | BM |
| Pulses | Pulses | Hard to digest | BD, BM |
| | Beans | Hard to digest | BD, BM, HT |
| | Chickpeas | Hard to digest | BD, BM, HT |

*Source:* Focus groups in three provinces.
*Note:* BD = Badakhshan; BM = Bamyan; HT = Herat.

perceived harmful effects. Eggs prepared by scrambling rather than frying or boiling (not in the shell) may be more acceptable because the form of the egg is less discernible to the child. Scrambled eggs may also be mixed in with other dishes (such as rice) and disguised. If local views are firm about eggs being harmful to speech development, then promote egg consumption after the child learns to speak.

- Explore modes of preparation of meats and pulses that would be more acceptable for infants and young children. Softer preparations may be easier to digest than food prepared for adults. Tenderizing meat and cooking it thoroughly to the point that it may be loose and stringy, and thus easy for young children to eat in small amounts, may be more acceptable. Mashing pulses, for example, could make them into a softer, safer food. Women commented that this suggestion was feasible. Pulses were consumed year-round.

- Nuts are not discussed as either beneficial or harmful, most likely because they are not associated with children's diets. However, nuts crushed into small sizes, powders, or butters could be added to children's foods to make them richer in protein.

## Beliefs about Fruits and Vegetables for Infants and Young Children

Beliefs about fruits and vegetables are summarized in table C.3. Comments and recommendations are as follows:

- Increase awareness about the benefits of fruits and vegetables for the nutrition and health of infants and young children, taking into consideration local concerns about harmful effects. Awareness in Herat was especially low. Mention the benefits of specific fruits and vegetables because food beliefs are associated with specific foods.
- Raisins were deemed acceptable and "good for blood" in Bamyan, which facilitates promoting them as an iron source for infants and young children.[1] Raisins cooked in *palaw* (a rice dish) are often soft and easy to eat. Raisins could also be mashed after cooking for children to avoid choking hazards.
- Digestibility and safety of foods (for example, food hygiene to prevent worm infections) are important considerations when promoting fruits and vegetables. Include food safety guidelines with fruit and vegetable promotion.
- Avoid promoting onions and hot peppers for young children because these vegetables are viewed as harmful for children in some areas and nutritional benefits are not significant at this age. Antimicrobial factors

**Table C.3    Beliefs about Fruits and Vegetables for Infants and Young Children**

| Food group | Food item | Belief | Province |
|---|---|---|---|
| *Beneficial* | | | |
| Fruits | Raisins | Energetic, good for blood | BM |
| Vegetables | Vegetables | Produce energy, contain vitamins | BD |
| *Harmful* | | | |
| Fruits | Fruits | Cause incontinence, diarrhea | BD |
| | Apples | Hard to digest | HT |
| | Apricots | Cause stomach problems | BD |
| | Melons | Harmful, hard to digest | HT |
| Vegetables | Vegetables | Difficult to digest, cause worms | BM, HT |
| | Cucumbers | Harmful, hard to digest | HT |
| | Eggplant | Harmful, hard to digest | HT |
| | Hot peppers | Not good for baby | BM |
| | Okra | Harmful, hard to digest | HT |
| | Onion | Not good for baby | BM |

*Source:* Focus groups in three provinces.
*Note:* BD = Badakhshan; BM = Bamyan; HT = Herat.

are associated with these foods, but other protective measures (for example, hygiene) would be more important to emphasize.

## Note

1. Research in Balkh province also identified raisins as good for blood (Levitt and others 2009).

## Reference

Levitt, Emily J., Rebecca J. Stoltzfus, David L. Pelletier, and Alice N. Pell. 2009. "A Community Food System Analysis as Formative Research for a Comprehensive Anemia Control Program in Northern Afghanistan." *Food Security* 1 (2): 177–95.

# Summary of Services Provided through the Ministry of Public Health Basic Package of Health Services

**Seven Elements of the Basic Package of Health Services and Their Components**

| | |
|---|---|
| 1. Maternal and newborn care | 1. Prenatal care |
| | 2. Delivery care |
| | 3. Postpartum care |
| | 4. Family planning |
| | 5. Care of the newborn |
| 2. Child health and immunization | 1. Expanded Programme on Immunization |
| | 2. Integrated Management of Childhood Illness |
| 3. Public nutrition | 1. Prevention of malnutrition |
| | 2. Assessment of malnutrition |
| 4. Communicable disease treatment and control | 1. Control of tuberculosis |
| | 2. Control of malaria |
| | 3. Prevention of HIV and AIDS |
| 5. Mental health | 1. Mental health education and awareness |
| | 2. Case identification and treatment |
| 6. Disability and physical rehabilitation services | 1. Disability awareness, prevention, and education |
| | 2. Provision of physical rehabilitation services |
| | 3. Case identification, referral, and follow-up |
| 7. Regular supply of essential drugs | 1. List of all essential drugs needed |

*Source:* Draft of revised policy document, 2010.

# Nutrition Components of the Basic Package of Health Services

| | Health facility level | | | | | |
|---|---|---|---|---|---|---|
| Interventions and services provided | Health post | Health subcenter | Basic health center | Mobile health team | Comprehensive health center | District hospital |
| **Assessment of malnutrition (population level)** | | | | | | |
| Nutritional status | Estimate prevalence of malnutrition—z-score using indexes of weight for height (wasting), weight for age (underweight), and height for age (stunting)—as well as the underlying causes. Surveys are conducted at the district or provincial level for purposes of baseline, monitoring, and evaluation or in case of obvious deterioration in nutritional situation. | | | | | |
| **Prevention of malnutrition** | | | | | | |
| Vitamin A supplementation for children 6–9 months | Yes, during National Immunization Days (NIDs) | No; yes after NIDs stop | No; yes after NIDs stop | No; yes after NIDs stop | No; yes after NIDs stop | No; yes after NIDs stop |
| Promotion of iodized salt | Yes | Yes | Yes | Yes | Yes | Yes |
| Promotion of balanced micronutrient-rich foods | Yes | Yes | Yes | Yes | Yes | Yes |
| Support and promotion of exclusive breastfeeding | Yes | Yes | Yes | Yes | Yes | Yes |
| Promotion of appropriate complementary feeding for young children with behavior changes | Yes | Yes | Yes | Yes | Yes | Yes |
| Community food demonstration | Yes | Yes | Yes | Yes | Yes | Yes |
| Growth monitoring and promotion for less than 2 years[a] (where applicable and linked with Integrated Management of Childhood Illness) | Yes | Yes | Yes | Yes | Yes | Yes |
| Iron and folic acid supplementation for pregnant and lactating women | Yes | Yes | Yes | Yes | Yes | Yes |
| Vitamin A supplementation postpartum | Yes | Yes | Yes | Yes | Yes | Yes |

| | | | | | |
|---|---|---|---|---|---|
| Promotion of maternal nutritional status[b] | Yes | Yes | Yes | Yes | Yes |
| Control and prevention of diarrheal disease and parasitic infections | Yes | Yes | Yes | Yes | Yes |
| Based on analysis of causes of malnutrition, support and advocacy for interventions to address underlying causes | Basic Package of Health Services nongovernmental organizations demonstrate an understanding of underlying causes and outline appropriate interventions to prevent and address malnutrition, including in areas of food security, social and care environment, and health (including water and sanitation). | | | | |

*Treatment of malnutrition*

| | | | | | |
|---|---|---|---|---|---|
| Micronutrient deficiency diseases diagnosis and treatment | Identify and refer | Yes | Yes | Yes | Yes |
| Treatment of severe malnutrition based on Ministry of Public Health protocols for 24-hour care for phase I, day care or home treatment for phase II, and follow-up[c] | No, refer | Prereferral treatment and refer | Prereferral treatment and refer | Prereferral treatment and refer | Prereferral treatment and refer |
| Treatment of severe malnutrition at community therapeutic centers[d]: community mobilization and screening | Yes, refer | Prereferral treatment and refer | Yes | Yes | Yes |
| Outpatient management | No | Yes | Yes | Yes | Yes |
| Inpatient care and stabilization center | No | No | No | No | Yes |
| Treatment of moderate malnutrition only if acute malnutrition levels higher than 10% with additional risk factors | No | Where applicable | No | No | No |

*(continued)*

| Interventions and services provided | Health post | Health subcenter | Basic health center | Mobile health team | Comprehensive health center | District hospital |
|---|---|---|---|---|---|---|
| **Surveillance and referral** | | | | | | |
| Clinic-based surveillance: all children under 5 years old measured for weight for height (using health management information system forms), trends monitored, and children showing developmental delay referred to physiotherapy services | No | Yes | Yes | Yes | Yes | No |
| Screening and referral of at-risk patients using mid-upper-arm circumference, weight and height, or clinical signs of micronutrient deficiency diseases | Yes | Yes | Yes | Yes | Yes | Yes |

*Source:* Ministry of Public Health.

*Note:* a. During 2004 or 2005, the Ministry of Public Health, in collaboration with the World Health Organization, carried out an assessment to identify what needs (resources, training, skills, and adaptation) should be in place for effective growth monitoring and promotion in Afghanistan. As indicated in the infant and young child feeding strategic plan and the Public Nutrition Policy and Strategy, approaches to growth promotion that have proven successful elsewhere will be adapted for each level and tested in the Afghan situation before careful scaling up.

b. Improving the nutritional status of women remains a priority, but a strategy for addressing the poor nutritional status of women is still being developed.

c. The Ministry of Public Health currently has guidelines and a strategy to support hospital-based (24-hour and day care) treatment.

d. Community therapeutic centers with their components will be implemented where vertical input is provided by the United Nations Children's Fund in agreement with the Public Nutrition Department.

# The Afghanistan National Development Strategy Structure

| Security | Governance | | Social and economical development | | | | | |
|---|---|---|---|---|---|---|---|---|
| Pillar 1 | Pillar 2 | Pillar 3 | Pillar 4 | Pillar 5 | Pillar 6 | Pillar 7 | Pillar 8 |
| 1. Security | 2. Good governance | 3. Infrastructure and natural resources | 4. Education and culture | 5. Health and nutrition | 6. Agriculture and rural development | 7. Social protection | 8. Economic governance and private sector development |

**Sectors**

| Security | Justice | Energy | Education | Health and nutrition | Agriculture and rural development | Social protection | Private sector development and trade |
|---|---|---|---|---|---|---|---|
| | Governance, public administrative reform, and human rights | Transportation | Culture, media, and youth | | | Refugees, returnees and internal displayed persons | |
| | Religious affairs | Water resource management | | | | | |
| | | Information and communications technology | | | | | |
| | | Urban development | | | | | |
| | | Mining | | | | | |

Cross-cutting issues
Capacity building
Gender equity
Counternarcotics
Regional cooperation
Anticorruption
Environment
*Nutrition?*

*Source:* Government of Afghanistan.

# Organizational Chart of Ministry of Public Health's Public Nutrition Department (under Preventive Medicine)

**High Counsel**

**Executive Board**

**Advisory Board**

**Bioethical Board**

**Adviser**

**Minister of Public Health**

### Deputy Minister for Technical Affairs

**Afghan Public Health Institute GD**
- Public Health Research Directorate
- Ghazanfar Institute of Health Sciences Dir
- P H and Management Training Dept
- Surveillance/DEWS Department
- Healthy Behaviour Promotion Dept
- P H Laboratories Dept
- Food and Drug Quality Control Laboratories Dept
- Informatics and Advanced IT Unit

- Legislation Implementation Ensuring Dept
- Forensic Medicine Dir
- Food and Drug Control Dept
- Internal Audit
- Pharmacy Enterprises

**Policy and Planning GD**
- Planning Dept
- M and E and QA Directorate
- Foreign Aid Coordination and HCF Directorate
- Health Care Financing Dept
- Construction Planning and Supervision Dept
- HMIS Unit

### Deputy Minister for Health Care Services Provision

**Health Care Services Provision GD**

- Preventive Basic Health Care Directorate
- BPHS Dept
- Environmental Health Dept
- Mental Health Dept
- EPI Dept
- Public Nutrition Dept
- Drug Demand Reduction Unit
- Prevention of Blindness Unit
- Dentistry Unit
- Nomads Health Unit
- CDC Directorate
- TB Dept
- Malaria and Leishmaniasis Dept
- HIV/AIDS Unit
- Emergency Preparedness and Response Dept

- Curative and Diagnostic Facilities Dept
- EPHS Dept
- Nursing Dept
- Central Blood Bank
- Radiology Dept
- Disability and Rehabilitation Unit
- Private Facilities Unit
- Central Hospitals Directorate
- RH Directorate
- SMI Dept
- Family Planning Dept
- Gender Unit
- Child and Adolescent Health Directorate
- Adolescent Health Dept
- School Health Unit
- IMCI Unit

### Deputy Minister for Administrative Affairs

**Pharmaceutical Affairs GD**
- Medicine Information and Devt Drug Affairs Directorate
- Drug Institutions Establishment Dept
- Drug Planning Dept
- Drug Preparation and Registration Dept
- Controlled Drugs Dept

**Administration GD**
- Deputy Admin. Dir
- Finance and Accounting Dir
- Procurement Dir
- Central Stock Dept
- Central Workshop Dept
- Transport Unit
- Maintenance Unit

**Human Resource GD**
- Clinical Specialization Dept
- Personnel Management Dept
- Reform Implementation and Capacity Building Management Dept
- Office of the Minister
- Documents and Archive Unit
- Public Relation Dept
- Provincial Health Liaison Dept
- International Relations Dept
- Secretariat of Boards
- Spokesman

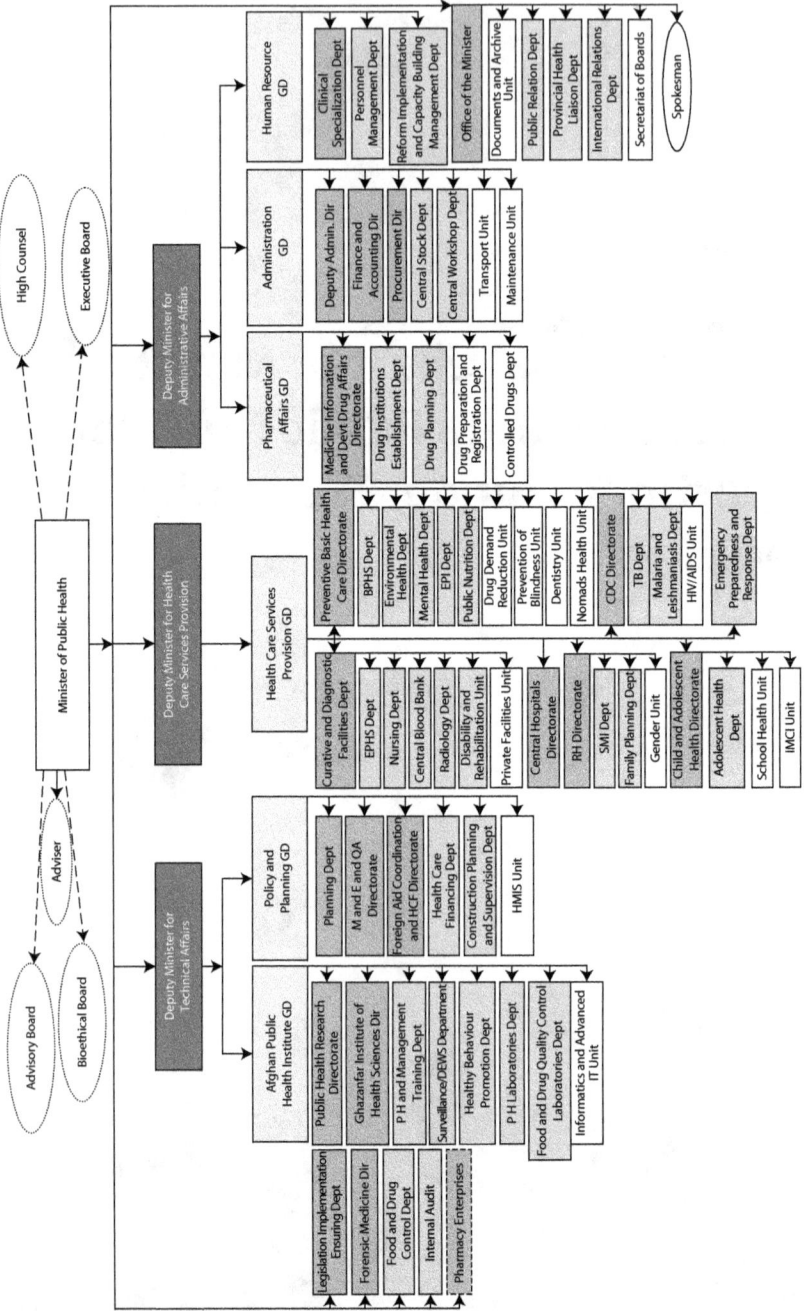

*Source:* Ministry of Public Health.

# Organizational Chart of the Ministry of Agriculture, Irrigation, and Livestock

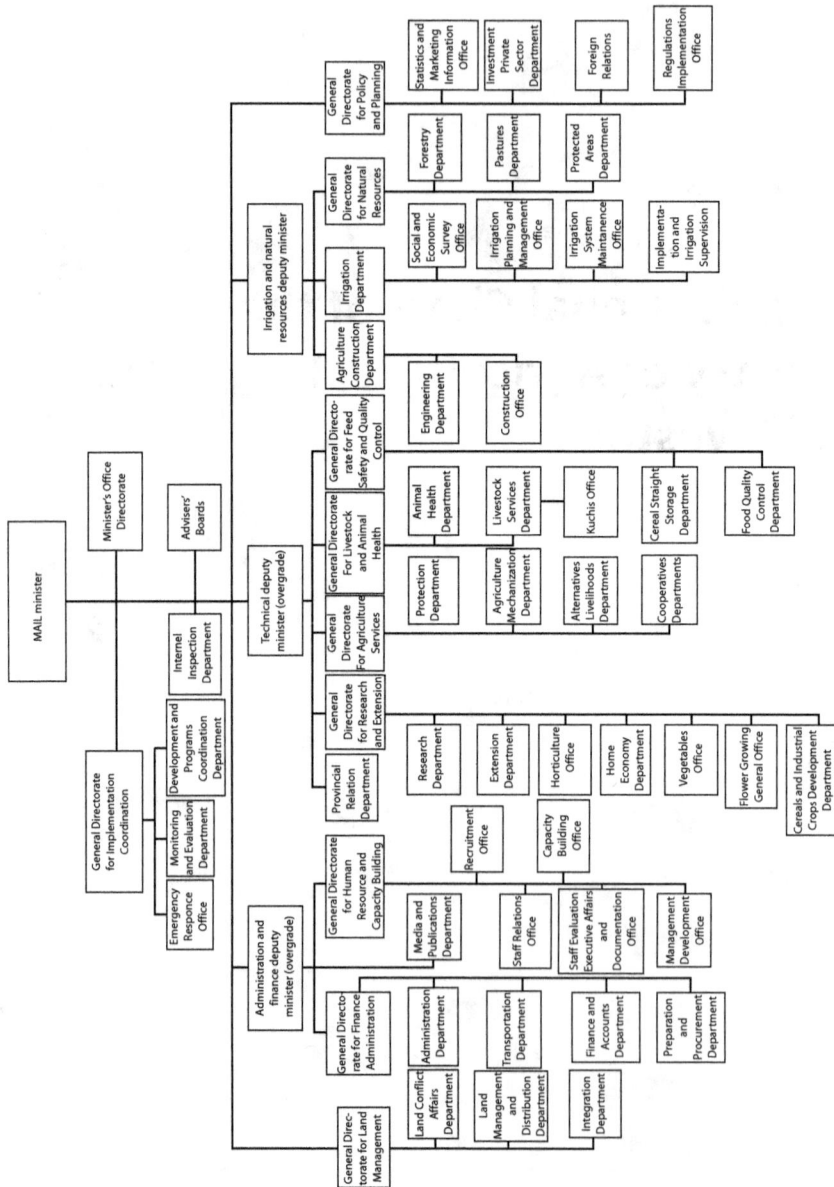

**MAIL minister**

- Minister's Office Directorate
- Advisers' Boards

General Directorate for Implementation Coordination
- Emergency Response Office
- Monitoring and Evaluation Department
- Development and Programs Coordination Department
- Internal Inspection Department

**Technical deputy minister (overgrade)**

**Irrigation and natural resources deputy minister**

**Administration and finance deputy minister (overgrade)**

General Directorate for Policy and Planning
- Statistics and Marketing Information Office
- Investment Private Sector Department
- Foreign Relations
- Regulations Implementation Office

General Directorate for Natural Resources
- Forestry Department
- Pastures Department
- Protected Areas Department
- Social and Economic Survey Office
- Irrigation Planning and Management Office
- Irrigation System Maintenance Office
- Implementation and Irrigation Supervision

Irrigation Department

Agriculture Construction Department

General Directorate for Feed Safety and Quality Control
- Engineering Department
- Construction Office

General Directorate For Livestock and Animal Health
- Animal Health Department
- Livestock Services Department
- Kuchis Office
- Cereal Straight Storage Department
- Food Quality Control Department

General Directorate For Agriculture Services
- Protection Department
- Agriculture Mechanization Department
- Alternatives Livelihoods Department
- Cooperatives Departments

General Directorate for Research and Extension
- Research Department
- Extension Department
- Horticulture Office
- Home Economy Department
- Vegetables Office
- Flower Growing General Office
- Cereals and Industrial Crops Development Department

Provincial Relation Department

General Directorate for Human Resource and Capacity Building
- Media and Publications Department
- Recruitment Office
- Staff Relations Office
- Capacity Building Office
- Staff Evaluation Executive Affairs and Documentation Office
- Management Development Office

General Directorate for Finance Administration
- Administration Department
- Transportation Department
- Finance and Accounts Department
- Preparation and Procurement Department

General Directorate for Land Management
- Land Conflict Affairs Department
- Land Management and Distribution Department
- Integration Department

*Source:* Ministry of Agriculture, Irrigation, and Livestock.

*Note:* The Home Economics Department is under the technical deputy minister of the General Directorate for Research and Extension.

# Job Description for Provincial Nutrition Officers

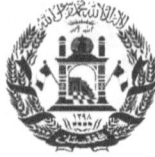

Islamic Republic of Afghanistan
Ministry of Public Health
Provincial Health Directorate

JOB DESCRIPTION: November 20, 2008

| | |
|---|---|
| Title of position: | Provincial Nutrition Officer |
| Department: | Provincial Health Unit |
| Location: | Province center |
| Report to: | Provincial Health Director |
| Subordinates: | None |
| Grade: | 3 |

**Scope of work:** All nutrition and nutrition-related medical activities at the province level in line with the Ministry of Public Health (MOPH) Public Nutrition Policy

**Purpose:**

(i) The overall coordination of public nutrition activities, at the province level, with relevant departments in the Provincial Health Unit, Public Nutrition Department of the MOPH, relevant line ministries in the province, and other partner organizations.

(ii) Support, facilitate, and monitor the implementation and integration of public nutrition interventions at the provincial level and district level, in line with MOPH policies, guidelines, and protocols.

**Responsibilities:**
**A. Assessment and analysis**

- Understand the extent and severity of malnutrition in the province and the underlying causes.
- Participate in surveys with technical support from the MOPH or partner organization where applicable.

- Support training of survey enumerators where applicable.
- Compile records of all surveys conducted in the area and forward copies to the central MOPH.
- Undertake rapid assessment in collaboration with the MOPH and/or partners.
- Supervise and analyze clinic-based surveillance in collaboration with the Health Management Information System (HMIS) Officer at the comprehensive health center (CHC) and basic health center (BHC) levels.
- Supervise and analyze nutritional screening information at the health post level.

**B. Support implementation and integration of public nutrition related activities**

a) Support implementation and integration of nutritional activities and strengthening Basic Package of Health Services (BPHS) regarding prevention and treatment of malnutrition (for example, information, education, and communication messages, vitamin A supplementation, maternal nutrition, infant and young child feeding, control of diarrheal diseases, micronutrient deficiency disease referral and treatment, moderate and severe malnutrition referral and treatment, etc.).
b) Support implementation of complementary provincial interventions where applicable.
  - Support installation and functioning of salt factories.
  - Support Baby-Friendly Hospital Initiative.
  - Support Therapeutic Feeding Unit (TFU) Training Centers at provincial level.
  - Support decentralized fortification of flour.

c) Support the activities of Community Health Workers (CHWs) through training and technical support.

**C. Monitor interventions and ensure high quality of services**

- Supervise, monitor, and evaluate public nutrition activities at all levels of service delivery, specifically:
- Monitor and support hospital-based TFUs for treatment of severe malnutrition according to MOPH Public Nutrition Guidelines.
- Monitor and support community-based Management of Acute Malnutrition for treatment of acute malnutrition according to MOPH Public Nutrition Guidelines.

- Monitor salt iodization program (production level, market and household levels).
- Collect and analyze of MOPH public nutrition monitoring forms for Supplementary Feeding Programs (SFPs), conduct monitoring visits of SFPs, and give feedback.
- Monitor food stocks in hospitals.
- Monitor quality of food aid programs.
- Monitor other public nutrition–related activities as directed by MOPH Public Nutrition Department.
- Promote and support optimal infant and young child feeding and care practices through monitoring of implementation of Code of Marketing of Breast Milk Substitutes and general nutrition communication.

**D. Conduct training and support capacity development at all levels of health facility and feedback**

a) At all four levels of facilities (hospital, CHC, BHC, and health post)
- Conduct trainings for CHWs, provincial MOPH staff, and staff of related ministries on specific modules prepared by the MOPH Public Nutrition Department (SFPs, Hospital-Based Management and Treatment of Severe Malnutrition, and others as developed).
- Conduct trainings for CHWs, provincial MOPH staff, and staff of related ministries on MOPH Public Nutrition Guidelines on micronutrient deficiency diseases (and other guidelines as developed).

b) Collect, compile, analyze, and use public nutrition data, and provide timely feedback to MOPH Public Nutrition Kabul as well as the implementing organization.
c) Travel in the field at least one week per month; submit a mission report to the Provincial Health Director of each trip.

**E. Coordination of all food and nutrition interventions and raising awareness of public nutrition and reporting**

- Develop and maintain simple database of SFPs, TFUS, food aid, and BPHS using framework.
- Maintain inventory of areas of operation and types of nutrition-related programming and share information with concerned organizations (for example, World Food Programme on food commodity distribution).

- Conduct nutrition coordination meeting once every three months.
- Participate in the Provincial Coordination Committee (PCC) meetings.
- Ensure that organizations are aware of and familiar with MOPH public nutrition policies, protocols, guidelines, strategies, and activities as well as BPHS.
- Provide three quarterly activity reports and one annual activity report to the Provincial Health Director.

## Qualifications:

- University qualification (does not necessarily have to be a medical degree)
- Experience in public health programs
- Highly motivated
- Dari and Pashto languages (written and spoken)
- Strong analytical skills
- Ability to travel widely within the province
- Excellent communication and interpersonal skills
- Ability to think broadly beyond narrow technical interventions
- Basic computer skills; MS Word
- English language preferable

## Specific outputs over the next 12 months:

- Simple database created that tracks areas of operation and types of nutrition-related programs to determine areas of need and gaps in coverage
- Records kept of surveys and surveillance data collected and sent to the central level
- Regular participation in PCC meetings
- Facilitation of four nutrition coordination meetings at provincial level
- Working partnership developed with HMIS Officer, including facilitating training of performance-based partnership agreement (PPA) nongovernment organization (NGO) in new HMIS forms
- At least 12 visits to the field and report of findings distributed
- Regular monitoring visits and reports of findings on nutrition-related programming generated, shared at the provincial level through the PCC and central level through reporting (e.g., SFPs, TFUs, salt factories, Baby-Friendly Hospitals, flour fortification factories, hospital food stocks, etc.)

- Facilitation of initial training and refresher training of MOPH staff, PPA NGO, CHWs and health facility staff in MOPH policies and guidelines
- Provision of updates on development in MOPH Public Nutrition Guidelines to provincial MOPH and NGOs as they are received

**Performance indicators:**

- Three quarterly and one annual report have been submitted to the Provincial Health Director
- At least six nutrition coordination meetings at the province level have been organized, chaired by the Provincial Nutrition Officer, and minutes of its meetings are available.
- At least 12 weeks have been spent in the field the past months, and mission reports of trips are available.
- Three quarterly and one annual report have been drafted and submitted to the Provincial Health Director.

**Appraisal process:** The Provincial Nutrition Officer will be appraised by the Provincial Health Director after three months, one year, and six-monthly thereafter using an MOPH standard appraisal format.

# Assessment of Capacity in Government Entities Responsible for Nutrition

This appendix assesses the capacity of the two main government of Afghanistan entities responsible for nutrition policies and programs: the Public Nutrition Department (PND) of the Ministry of Public Health (MOPH) and the Home Economics Department (HED) of the Ministry of Agriculture, Irrigation, and Livestock (MAIL). The methodology used is described by Potter and Brough (2004). This assessment uses a four-tier hierarchy of capacity-building needs: (a) structures, systems, and roles; (b) staff and facilities; (c) skills; and (d) tools. The first tier forms the base of the capacity structure, with each successive tier building on the previous one. Table J.1 provides information about the capacity elements within each tier.

## The MOPH's PND

This section discusses various aspects of the PND's capacity for nutrition policies, strategies, and programs.

### Structural Capacity

The PND is weakly positioned in the MOPH structure (appendix G). Decision-making forums exist (for example, task forces and consultative groups) where intersectoral discussions may occur. However, if corporate

**Table J.1  Nine Elements of Systemic Capacity Building**

| Component | Description |
|---|---|
| *Tier 1: Structures, systems, and roles* | |
| Structural capacity | Do decision-making forums exist where intersectoral discussions can occur and decisions can be made, records can be kept, and individuals can be called to account for nonperformance? |
| Systems capacity | Do the flows of information, money, and managerial decisions function in a timely and effective manner? Can purchases be made without lengthy delays for authorization? Are proper filing and information systems in use? Are staffing arrangements and changes made in acceptable ways? Can private sector services be engaged as required? Is communication with the community good? Are sufficient links with other implementers (that is, nongovernment organizations) in place? |
| Role capacity | This element applies to individuals, teams, and structures such as committees. Have they been given the authority and responsibility to make the decisions essential to effective performance, whether regarding schedules, money, staff appointments, or the like? |
| *Tier 2: Staff and facilities* | |
| Workload capacity | Do enough staff members have broad enough skills to cope with the workload? Are job descriptions practical? Is the skill mix appropriate? |
| Supervisory capacity | Are reporting and monitoring systems in place? Are the lines of accountability clear? Can supervisors physically monitor their staffs? Are effective incentives and sanctions available? |
| Facility capacity | Are facilities big enough with the right staff in sufficient numbers? Are staff supports sufficient (offices, workshops, warehouses, and so forth) to support the workload? |
| Support-service capacity | Are facilities, training institutions, supply organizations, building services, administrative staff, research facilities, quality control services, and so on available to support the work? |
| *Tier 3: Skills* | |
| Personnel capacity | Is the staff sufficiently knowledgeable, skilled, and confident to perform properly? Do staff members need training, experience, or motivation? Are they deficient in technical skills, managerial skills, interpersonal skills, gender-sensitivity skills, or specific role-related skills? |
| *Tier 4: Tools* | |
| Performance capacity | Are the tools, money, equipment, consumables, and so on available to do the job? |

*Source:* Potter and Brough 2004.

decisions are made, the PND has no real authority over partners to enforce agreements pertaining to nutrition. As a result, nonperforming partners are rarely called to account. Accountability measures are informal and are based on the strength of personal networks within the nutrition community.

### Systems Capacity
The flows of information function in a timely manner when communication tools (for example, Internet, telephone, transportation) are adequate. The frequently limited availability of communication tools hampers information flow between the PND and its provincial officers as well as hampering communication with the nutrition community at large. Financial flows are delayed because of a lengthy procurement process through the Ministry of Finance. Private sector services cannot be contracted as needed (for example, to assist with policy revision between 2006 and 2008) because the PND hardly has a core budget. Decisions to support PND activities depend on the will and agendas of partners, despite PND advocacy. Managerial decision-making systems are satisfactory and decentralized, although staff members request additional training in management skills, given their largely clinical training as physicians.

### Role Capacity
Financial arrangements disempower the PND because the authority over use of funds is dictated by development partners. One currently pressing issue is the low rate for daily subsistence allowances for staff members who need to travel. Current levels do not cover expenses, which leads to decreased attendance at PND activities, trainings, and workshops.

### Workload Capacity
Staff members receive in-service and short-course training sessions that equip them to implement existing programs although they have no formal degree certification in nutrition. Development partners, such as the Food and Agriculture Organization of the United Nations (FAO), Micronutrient Initiative, United Nations Children's Fund, World Food Programme, and World Health Organization, often provide strong technical support for programs because all activities generally require outside support. Technical support is routinely requested for policy revision and other programmatic strategic planning activities. Sustained advocacy to mainstream nutrition in previous years has led to frequent invitations to

attend various coordination meetings. This "meeting overload" complicates schedules and makes meeting deadlines a challenge. Furthermore, the PND is experiencing difficulty retaining provincial and some national staff because of low salaries and inadequate operational support to complete functions of the job description.

### Supervisory Capacity

Reporting systems are in place between provincial and national officers, as are clear lines of accountability (management chains). However, the national staff faces challenges in monitoring the provincial staff because of communications and transportation difficulties. Security and severe weather conditions during parts of the year make in-country travel and communication problematic. The PND receives support from partners that fund projects for some monitoring activities. A lack of departmental transportation (owning a vehicle or renting a car and driver) hampers monitoring activities for both provincial and national staff members.

### Facility Capacity

Afghanistan has no training centers for nutrition. All training sessions are provided by independent consultants, the United Nations, and nongovernment organizations. The PND conducts nutrition training sessions with support from partners, but no separate institution is formally dedicated to nutrition training.

Therapeutic feeding units (TFUs) face a caseload greater than the facility can manage. Some PND staff members also noted that the logistical protocols for TFUs are not being followed because of space limitations in hospitals (see chapter 5 for details). Office space is also limited at national and provincial levels. Provincial nutrition officers in some provinces share a small office with another, unrelated health sector official. The PND has one main room with a large table in the center. This space is adequate for meetings of six to eight people, but the MOPH no longer has adequate space for larger training sessions, workshops, or presentations. The old meeting rooms have been converted into office space. Thus, the PND has had to rent space in hotel meeting rooms for recent workshops. Cultural norms have hindered women from attending meetings in hotels. A request was made for the renovation or building of new meeting spaces within the MOPH or a nearby government structure to facilitate women's involvement.

## Support-Service Capacity

As noted previously, the country has no training institutions or facilities for nutrition research. Some countries (for example, India, Peru, and Thailand) have established national nutrition institutes that support government policies and programs. Such an institute would be a valuable asset to Afghanistan's multisectoral nutrition system. Furthermore, the Afghanistan National Standards Authority, which is the regulatory body responsible for food safety and quality control (among other product safety activities), has potential to fulfill its given function, but it is weak in implementation capacity. Development partners are supportive to a degree that depends heavily on their own individual and institutional agendas. Long spans of time often elapse between hiring international employees because Afghanistan is a challenging and politically vulnerable environment.

## Personnel Capacity

Staff members have a growing knowledge base of nutrition programs under their leadership. However, as previously noted, technical skills for strategic planning, policy, research, advocacy, and general bureaucratic maneuvering are inadequate. Skills in supervising large-scale programs are weak. The MOPH's Human Resources Department questioned why five to seven PND staff members had not been supported to gain master's degrees abroad in nutrition. Distance learning for the national staff is of interest because no trained people are available to replace staff members who leave the country. More than five years has been invested in building the capacity of the PND staff members. Such training has led to increased confidence but dependence on these employees for nutrition within Afghanistan. Increased training would increase confidence to lead research and policy planning, among other functions. Motivation is also lacking in some respects because of low salaries. This lack of motivation manifests more as discouragement than as a lack of interest in performing the role. PND staff members request support for improving managerial, budgetary, and overall financial management skills as well.

## Performance Capacity

Partners have provided some supplies to assist with office work. However, these supplies are all linked to an activity or event. The PND has no core operating budget under its control. It has inadequate support for communications and transportation to maintain regular engagement with colleagues. In the TFUs, medicine supplies are reportedly often exhausted by midmonth, and there are delays in obtaining restocks. The TFUs also have an insufficient number of beds.

## Summary of Capacity Gaps of the MOPH PND

- Lack of formal training in nutrition and capacity development to manage large-scale programs
- Insufficient operational support for day-to-day activities and lack of a core budget permitting capacity to grow in financial management (that is, dependence on development partners for both large and small materials and need to get permission to draw funds for daily operational expenses)
- Lack of transportation (monthly car rental requested by national and provincial officers) for conducting standard operations, engaging with partners, and monitoring visits
- Lack of Internet and telephone communications to maintain contact with provincial officers and partners
- Space constraints impeding the involvement of women in PND activities
- Poor positioning of the PND within the MOPH operational chart, given the strategic importance of nutrition to national development objectives

## The MAIL's Home Economics Department

The same capacity assessment protocol was applied in the agriculture sector. The main department focusing on direct nutrition interventions is the MAIL's HED. The HED differs from the MOPH's PND in that FAO is an on-site partner, providing daily capacity-building support. (The PND began using this model between 2003 and 2005 when Tufts University consultants were posted in the MOPH to work side by side with the PND officers.)

### Structural Capacity

The HED participates or takes the lead with FAO in task forces and Afghanistan National Development Strategy consultative group meetings when it needs to consult with partners. In these meetings, corporate decisions can be made, but ability is limited to hold partners accountable to commitments related to nutrition or food security through existing structures. Collaborations succeed depending on the strengths of personal networks and relationships between organizational mandates.

### Systems Capacity

Support for the HED comes primarily from a German-funded FAO project. This project began in 2005 and was renewed after a three-year cycle through December 2010. This grant permits adequate communications and transportation, which facilitate flows of information and resources. Managerial decisions are made in a timely manner because bureaucracy between the national and provincial staffs is limited. Because the HED is the result of direct FAO support, private sector contractors may be hired if FAO approves. FAO does not have a core budget for projects and receives its funds through a proposal-writing process, which makes the HED very vulnerable after December 2010 because the MAIL has provided only limited support. The HED may be in the same situation as the MOPH PND is at present after December 2010.

### Role Capacity

The HED has moderate authority to make decisions essential to effective performance, and most important decisions are made together with FAO counterparts. Budget decisions are made together with FAO because all funds are earmarked for specific activities pursuant to the grant. In the absence of an FAO grant, the HED would be the main authority on nutrition and food security in the agriculture sector, but it would have a weak ability to take action without some core funding directly through the MAIL.

### Workload Capacity

Staff members are learning the skills required for their work in service and through study tours. FAO also provides numerous training sessions as well as day-to-day in-house capacity-building support for HED national officers. No HED officers have formal degree training in nutrition.

### Supervisory Capacity

National and provincial HED staff members communicate as they can. Communication limitations exist more at the provincial level—given the variable climate, security concerns, and cost of communications and transportation—than at the national level, where FAO provides logistical support. Project monitoring systems relate largely to participation and types of participation in HED activities rather than nutritional outcomes (for example, consumption).

### Facility Capacity

Facilities within the MAIL are adequate for the HED in Kabul, and larger spaces are available through MAIL or FAO offices. Provincial space varies but tends to be in the provincial MAIL department.

### Support Service Capacity

Some MAIL departments provide data supportive to nutrition policies and plans. This information relates to the food security surveillance mechanisms and data from other agriculture sector programs. Otherwise, FAO represents the main source of support to the HED.

### Personnel Capacity

As with the PND staff, the HED staff members are learning in service and through study tours. Staff members have a reasonable mastery of their project-related knowledge from multiple years of experience. However, technical support is still requested for strategic planning and policy, research, and program management. Navigating financial systems is also complex in the current aid environment.

### Performance Capacity

FAO supplies the HED's resources. As a result, the HED has the money and materials to conduct its programs. However, the HED does not operate at scale to the degree that it could, given the availability of trained staff members in 17 provinces. This lack of scale is limited by FAO funding and inadequate support from the development community.

### Gaps and Opportunities Related to the Capacity of the HED's Extension Office

- Ownership of activities related specifically to food security (apart from increased agricultural production and associated income generation) is weak at high levels of the MAIL and its development partners. Increased production and income generation do not directly translate into improved nutrition, especially for vulnerable household members (such as women, children, ill people, people with disabilities, or the elderly).
- The new National Agriculture Development Framework contains no explicit food security (or nutrition) policy (although the previous

master plan had a full chapter). Ongoing efforts are being pursued to mainstream food security and nutrition objectives into the core National Agriculture Development Framework programs.

- Available, trained HED staff members provide an opportunity to reach an additional 12 provinces (total 17) with infant and young child feeding and other household nutrition promotion activities.
- Without greater MAIL support, sustainability of HED activities is unclear beyond project funds provided by FAO, which end in December 2010.
- Formal nutrition training of HED staff members is needed through distance learning or courses abroad. Afghanistan currently has are no formal nutrition training programs.

## Reference

Potter, Christopher, and Richard Brough. 2004. "Systemic Capacity Building: A Hierarchy of Needs." *Health Policy and Planning* 19 (5): 336–54.

# Public Nutrition Partners According to the Type of Roles and Responsibilities

| Specific objective | Strategic components | Ministry of Public Health Departments | Other ministries | Technical and financial assistance providers | Implementing partners[a] |
|---|---|---|---|---|---|
| 1. Nutrition promotion | Harmonized nutrition promotion | HP, PND | MAIL, MOE, MORA, MOWA, MRRD | FAO, MI, UNICEF, USAID BASICS, WFP, WHO | BPHS NGOs, CHWs, DAIL, DOE, DOPH, DRRD, media, other NGOs, religious leaders, shuras |
| | Community based activities | CBHC, PND | MAIL, MOE, MORA, MOWA, MRRD | FAO, MI, UNICEF, USAID BASICS, WFP, WHO | BPHS NGOs, CHWs, FHAGs, literacy circles, NSP NGOs, producer groups, shuras |
| | Links to food security | PND | MAIL, MRRD | FAO, WFP | DAIL, DRRD, NGOs |
| 2. Infant and young child feeding | Advocacy, regulations, guidelines | PND, Policy and Planning | MOC, MOJ, MOWA | IBFAN, UNICEF, WABA, WHO | Emergency service providers, NGOs, private sector |
| | Community support | CBHC, PND | MAIL, MOE, MRRD | FAO, UNICEF, USAID BASICS, WHO | CHWs, FHAGs, literacy circles, NGOs (BPHS and others), producer groups, shuras |
| | Infant and young child feeding in BPHS and EPHS | CAH, CBHC, GCMU, HP, IMCI, PND, RH | | IBFAN, UNICEF, WABA, WHO | BPHS NGOs, CHWs |
| 3. Micronutrients | Universal salt iodization | Food and Drug Quality Control, PND | ANSA, MOC (customs houses), MOJ, MOMI, municipality | MI, UNICEF | Private sector: iodized salt producers, mine leasers, retailers, wholesalers; CHWs, media, NGOs, shuras |
| | Flour fortification | Food and Drug Quality Control, PND | ANSA, MAIL, MOC, MOJ | MI, WFP | Private sector: flour millers, retailers; CHWs, media, NGOs, shuras |
| | Ghee and oil fortification | Food and Drug Quality Control, PND | ANSA, MOC, MOJ | MI, UNICEF | Oil and ghee importers, retailers |
| | Complementary food fortification | Food and Drug Quality Control, PND | ANSA, MOC | MI, UNICEF | Private sector |
| | Supplementation | EPI, GCMU, PND | ANSA, MOC | FAO, MI, UNICEF, WHO | |

| | | | | |
|---|---|---|---|---|
| Nutrition education | HP, PND | MAIL, MRRD | FAO, MI, UNICEF, WHO | Media, NGOs, private sector |
| 4. Severe acute malnutrition | Screening | BPHS, CBHC, GCMU, PND | | UNICEF, WHO | BPHS NGOs, DOPH |
| | Inpatient care | BPHS, EPHS, GCMU, PND | | UNICEF, WHO | BPHS NGOs, DOPH |
| | Outpatient care | PND, BPHS | | UNICEF, WHO | BPHS NGOs |
| 5. Food safety | Consumer and food retailer education | IEC, Food and Drug Quality Control, PND | ANSA, MAIL, MOC | EU, FAO, USAID (MAIL), WHO | NGOs, private sector |
| | Food quality control system | Food and Drug Quality Control, PND | ANSA, MAIL, MOC | EU, FAO, UNIDO (ANSA), USAID (MAIL), WHO, World Bank | Private sector |
| 6. Nutrition Surveillance | Surveillance | HMIS, PND, third-party evaluation (JHU) | CSO, MAIL, MRRD | FAO, UNICEF, WFP, WHO | BPHS NGOs, CHWs, DOPH, JHU, NRVA |
| | Monitoring and evaluation | HMIS, Monitoring and Evaluation, PND, third-party evaluation (JHU) | CSO, MRRD | FAO, UNICEF, WFP, WHO | BPHS, DOPH, JHU, NRVA |
| 7. Nutrition in emergencies | Improved assessment and design | MOPH Emergency, PND | Disaster Management Committee, MAIL, MRRD | FAO, UNICEF, UN Office for Coordination of Humanitarian Assistance, WFP, WHO | DAIL, DOPH, DRRD, NGOs (BPHS and others) |
| | Food assistance | PND | Disaster Management Committee, MAIL, MRRD | WFP | DAIL, DOPH, DRRD, NGOs |

*(continued)*

| Specific objective | Strategic components | Ministry of Public Health Departments | Other ministries | Technical and financial assistance providers | Implementing partners[a] |
|---|---|---|---|---|---|
| | Management of Global Acute Malnutrition | PND | | FAO, MI, UNICEF, WFP, WHO | NGOs (BPHS and emergency service providers) |
| 8. Public nutrition capacity development | In-service training | HR, IMCI, PND | MAIL, MOE, MOWA, MRRD | FAO, MI, UNICEF, USAID BASICS, WFP, WHO | BPHS NGOs, other NGOs |
| | Preservice training | Health Sciences Institute, PND | Agriculture faculties, medical faculties, MOE, Ministry of Higher Education | FAO, MI, UNICEF, WFP, WHO | Agriculture faculties, medical universities, other technical assistance programs, supporting universities (University of Massachusetts Amherst) |
| | Strengthening of PND | General Directorate of Primary Health Care, HR, PND | | FAO, MI, UNICEF, USAID BASICS, WFP, WHO | |

*Source:* Authors' compilation.

*Note:* ANSA = Afghanistan National Standards Authority; BASICS = Basic Support for Institutionalizing Child Survival; BPHS = Basic Package of Health Services; CAH = Child and Adolescent Health; CBHC = Community-Based Health Care; CHW = community health worker; CSO = Central Statistics Office; DAIL = Department of Agriculture, Irrigation, and Livestock; DOE = Department of Education; DOPH = Department of Public Health; DRRD = Department of Rural Rehabilitation and Development; EPHS = Essential Package of Hospital Services; EPI = Expanded Programme on Immunization; EU = European Union; FAO = Food and Agriculture Organization; FHAG = family health action group; GCMU = Grants, Contracts, and Management Unit; HMIS = Health Management Information System; HP = Health Promotion; HR = Human Resources; IBFAN = International Baby Food Action Network; IEC = information, education, and communication; IMCI = Integrated Management of Childhood Illness; JHU = Johns Hopkins University; MAIL = Ministry of Agriculture, Irrigation, and Livestock; MI = Micronutrient Initiative; MOC = Ministry of Commerce; MOE = Ministry of Education; MOJ = Ministry of Justice; MOMI = Ministry of Mines and Industry; MORA = Ministry of Religious Affairs; MOWA = Ministry of Women's Affairs; MRRD = Ministry of Rural Rehabilitation and Development; NGO = nongovernment organization; NRVA = National Risk and Vulnerability Assessment; NSP = National Solidarity Program; PND = Public Nutrition Department; RH = Reproductive Health; UNICEF = United Nations Children's Fund; UNIDO = United Nations International Development Organization; USAID = U.S. Agency for International Development; WABA = World Alliance for Breastfeeding Action; WFP = World Food Programme; WHO = World Health Organization.

a. At the provincial level, the government ministries are renamed with "D" for department instead of "M" for ministry.

# Simple Growth Promotion Card Developed for Demonstration Project in Afghanistan (BASICS III Project)

Child's age: _____     Child's address: _____

Community health worker's name: _____     Mothers' support group name: _____

**Child's weight each month is marked on the picture of the scale.**

| agreement practiced by mother? | |
|---|---|
| | |
| | |
| | |
| | |
| | |
| | |
| | |
| | |
| | |
| | |

| agreement information | | |
|---|---|---|
| | | |
| | | |
| | | |
| | | |
| | | |
| | | |
| | | |
| | | |
| | | |

weight gain status

| date | | |
|---|---|---|
| | | |
| | | |
| | | |
| | | |
| | | |
| | | |
| | | |
| | | |
| | | |

BABY WEIGHING SCALE

TO WEIGH
25Kg x 100g
NOT LEGAL FOR TRADE

*Source:* United States Agency for International Development Basic Support for Institutionalizing Child Survival (BASICS) III Project.

# Overview of the Components of the Government Nutrition System in Afghanistan

**Private sector partnerships:** Flour fortification, USI exploration of multiple micronutrient powders for children and adults, vitamin A in oil or ghee imports, use weddings as an opportunity for distribution of iron and folic acid

**Ministry of Public Health**

**BPHS, EPHS**

**Public Nutrition Department**

- **Prenatal care** (iron and folic acid, breastfeeding counseling, USI)
- **Baby-Friendly Hospital Initiative** (breastfeeding counseling and support)
- **Postpartum** vitamin A
- **IMCI** (IYCF, USI, anemia control, zinc in diarrhea treatment, malaria control)
- **TFUs** (treatment of acute malnutrition)
- **SFP** if GAM >15%; full **CMAM** if GAM >10%, including multiple micronutrient powders
- **CHWs** (community-based growth promotion with family health action groups—pilot study; various functions related to health, hygiene, IYCF, USI, vitamin A through NIDs, referrals)
- vitamin A through **NIDs**
- **HMIS** surveillance (weight for height)

**Ministry of Agriculture, Irrigation, and Livestock**

**Home Economics Department (extension)**

- **Routine food security surveillance** during year for crop and price-level estimates (early warning systems)
- Trainings on **improved complementary feeding**
- **School-Based Nutrition Program**
- Household food security—food processing and preservation trainings for consumption and income generation
- **Horticulture and Livestock Project** as platform (for example, women's and men's producer groups, poultry, dairy)
- Cosignatory on Afghanistan National Development Strategy Health and Nutrition Strategy

**Ministry of Rural Rehabilitation and Development**

- Household-level food security surveillance nationwide every 2 years through **NRVA**
- **Safe drinking water**
- **Improved sanitation**
- **Hygiene education** (with many partners)
- Many community development programs available as **platforms for nutrition programming** (for example, National Solidarity Program, women's groups)

**Ministry of Higher Education:** Revision of curriculum in medical schools and some training centers for nutrition in 2010

**Joint Program for Nutrition** (with FAO, UNICEF, and WHO)

**Other contributing ministries**

**Ministry of Justice:** Oversight of legislation (for example, Code of Marketing of Breast Milk Substitutes; maternity laws, fortification)

**Ministry of Commerce:** Support for public-private partnerships (for example, fortification); also supports Afghanistan National Standards Authority for food safety and quality control

**Ministry of Education:** Partnering with MAIL on School-Based Nutrition Program; exploring links with Healthy Schools Initiative to scale up

**Ministry of Labor, Social Affairs, Martyrs, and Disabled:** Use of nutrition as an outcome indicator of social protection programs; welcoming of nutrition promotion through day care centers, orphanages, and kindergartens

**Ministry of Women's Affairs:** Provision of women's groups (for example, literacy) for nutrition promotion

**Ministry of Religious Affairs:** Promotion of nutrition to general public

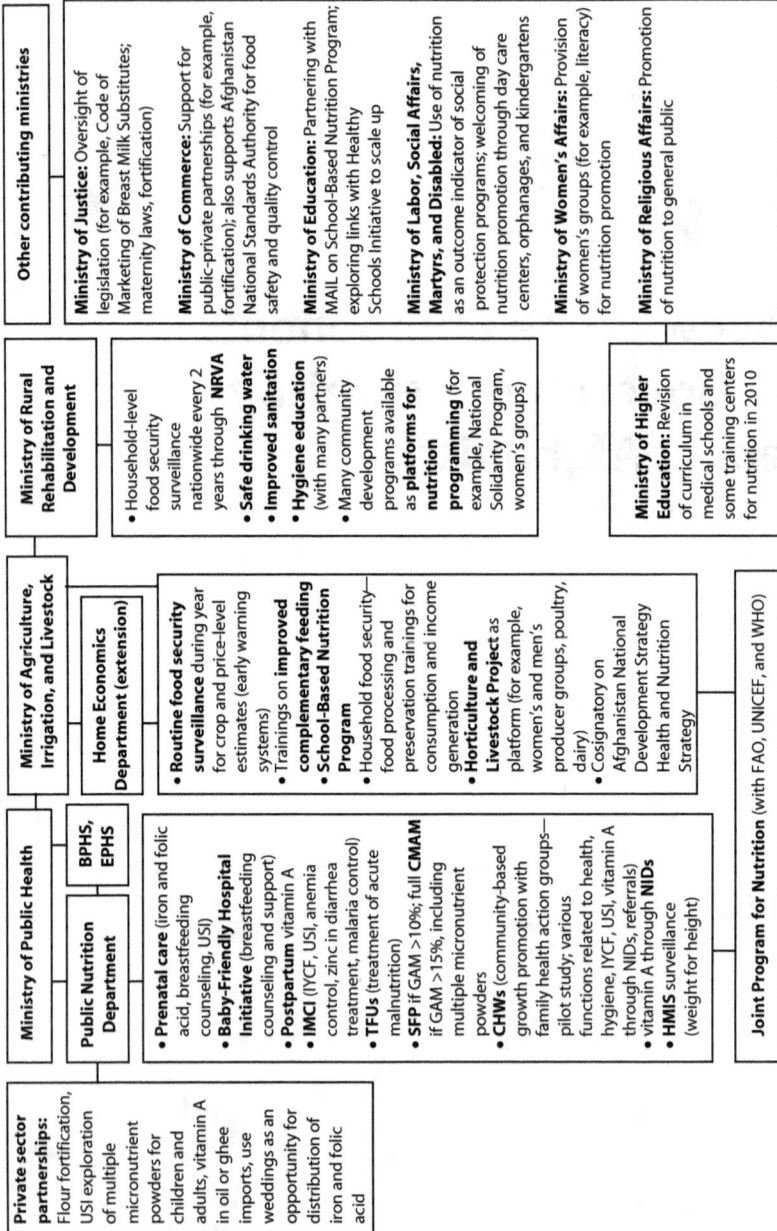

*Source:* Author compilation.

*Note:* BPHS = Basic Package of Health Services; CHW = community health worker; CMAM = Community-Based Management of Acute Malnutrition; EPHS = Essential Package of Hospital Services; FAO = Food and Agriculture Organization; GAM = global acute malnutrition; HMIS = Health Management Information System; IMCI = Integrated Management of Childhood Illness; IYCF = infant and young child feeding; NID = National Immunization Day; NRVA = National Risk and Vulnerability Assessment; SFP = supplemental feeding program; TFU = therapeutic feeding unit; UNICEF = United Nations Children's Fund; USI = universal salt iodization; WHO = World Health Organization.

# Glossary

Definitions here are derived from *Repositioning Nutrition as Central to Development* (World Bank 2006) unless otherwise stated. Malnutrition data are expressed using the new World Health Organization international references.

*Malnutrition:* A term that comprises all forms of "bad" nutrition, including overweight and obesity. The term *undernutrition* is therefore increasingly used to designate malnutrition that is due to a lack of food or nutrients. (Sometimes the term *malnutrition* is still used as an equivalent to *undernutrition*.) There are several forms of malnutrition:

- *Chronic undernutrition (or stunting):* Failure to reach linear growth potential because of inadequate nutrition or poor health. Chronic undernutrition implies long-term undernutrition and poor health and is measured as height for age that is two z-scores below the international reference. This measure is usually a good indicator of long-term undernutrition among young children. For children under the age of 12 months, recumbent length is used instead of height.

- *Acute undernutrition (or wasting):* Weight (in kilograms) divided by height (in meters squared) that is two z-scores below the international reference. Acute undernutrition describes a recent or current severe process leading to significant weight loss, usually a consequence of acute starvation or severe disease. It is commonly used as an indicator of undernutrition among children and is especially useful in emergency situations such as famine.

- *Underweight:* Low weight for age; that is, two z-scores below the international reference for weight for age. Underweight implies stunting or wasting and is an indicator of undernutrition.

- *Overweight:* Excess weight relative to height. Overweight is commonly measured by body mass index (BMI) among adults. The international reference for adults is as follows:
  - Grade I: 25.00–29.99 BMI (overweight)
  - Grade II: 30.00–39.99 BMI (obese)
  - Grade III: 40.00 or greater BMI

  For children, overweight is measured as weight for height that is two z-scores above the international reference.

- *Low birth weight (LBW):* Weight at birth below 2.5 kilograms. LBW babies are at higher risk of death and undernutrition and may have a wide range of disorders.

- *Chronic energy deficiency (CED):* The term that is used to designate adult undernutrition because of a lack of energy (as opposed to micronutrients). CED is indicated by weight loss and is measured using the body mass index.

- *Micronutrient deficiency disorders (MDDs):* Term encompassing a wide range of disorders that are due to an insufficient intake or use of vitamins or minerals. Different symptoms and disorders are associated with each deficiency. For example, iron deficiency can cause anemia; iodine deficiency can cause mental impairment, goiter, and cretinism; vitamin A deficiency leads to increased child mortality and night blindness; and vitamin C deficiency causes scurvy. Each deficiency can cause a range of symptoms according to the severity of the deficiency, and many MDDs are associated with an increased risk of morbidity.

*Anemia:* Low level of hemoglobin in the blood, as evidenced by a reduced quality or quantity of red blood cells. Fifty percent of anemia worldwide is caused by iron deficiency.

*Body mass index (BMI):* Body weight in kilograms divided by height in meters squared ($kg/m^2$). BMI is used as an index of "fatness." Both high BMI (overweight = BMI greater than 25.0) and low BMI (thinness = BMI less than 18.5) are considered inadequate.

*z-score:* The deviation of an individual's value from the median value of a reference population, divided by the standard deviation of the reference population.

The following definitions of infant and young child feeding (IYCF) practices are from Afghanistan's National IYCF Strategy for 2009 (MOPH 2009).

*Early initiation of breastfeeding:* Breastfeeding within the first hour of birth. Early initiation of breastfeeding is recommended so that infants receive the "first milk" (*colostrum*), which is rich in immunological factors and nutrients required by the neonate. Colostrum is available to the child only during the first days postpartum.

*Exclusive breastfeeding (birth to six months):* A breast milk–only diet for the infant during the first six months of life. Other liquids (such as water, tea, juices, and ritual liquids) and solid and semisolid foods are to be avoided. Exclusive breastfeeding has been shown to be associated with a reduced incidence of diarrhea, respiratory infections, and allergies. Promotion of exclusive breastfeeding is a key child survival strategy in resource-poor countries (WHO Collaborative Study Team 2000).

*Continued breastfeeding (until two years):* Breastfeeding until the child is two years old. Continued breastfeeding at a sustained high level at least for the first year and continued breastfeeding until age two years and beyond are beneficial for both infants' nutrition and mothers' lactational amenorrhea (cessation of menses during lactation), a natural method of birth spacing. The Holy Qur'an recommends breastfeeding for two years.

*Appropriate complementary feeding:* Introduction of solid and semisolid foods. Children 6 to 24 months old are to continue breastfeeding, with the addition of nutritionally adequate, safe, and appropriate complementary foods until age two years during their transition to the family diet (WHO 2001). These first foods are termed *complementary* because they are to be given as a complement (addition) to breast milk. After the age of six months, breast milk provides some but not all of the nutrients a child needs for healthy growth and development, and the child requires additional foods from the family food supply. Complementary feeding is essential to provide growing infants nutrients (specifically, iron, zinc, vitamin A, energy, and protein) that are in insufficient quantities in breast milk to meet the child's nutrient requirements for health, growth, and development. *Note:* Complementary foods should not replace breastfeeding as a source of nourishment for the child. They are therefore not "weaning" foods and should not be referred to as such, because children are encouraged to fully continue breastfeeding during this period. These foods are also different from supplementary foods (that is, foods given to a sick child for a short period of time from sources outside the household as a therapeutic treatment).

*Breast milk substitute (BMS):* Any food being marketed or otherwise represented as a partial or total replacement for breast milk, whether or not suitable for that purpose. BMSs include infant formula; other milk products; therapeutic milk; bottle-fed complementary foods marketed for children up to two years of age; and complementary foods, juices, and teas marketed for infants under six months of age.

## References

MOPH (Ministry of Public Health). 2009. *National Infant and Young Child Feeding Strategy*. Kabul: MOPH.

WHO (World Health Organization). 2001. "Guiding Principles for Complementary Feeding of the Breastfed Child." WHO, Geneva.

WHO (World Health Organization) Collaborative Study Team on the Role of Breastfeeding on the Prevention of Infant Mortality. 2000. "Effect of Breastfeeding on Infant and Child Mortality Due to Infectious Diseases in Less Developed Countries: A Pooled Analysis." *Lancet* 355 (9202): 451–55.

World Bank. 2006. *Repositioning Nutrition as Central to Development: A Strategy for Large-Scale Action*. Washington, DC: World Bank.

# Index

Page numbers followed by *n* refer to numbered notes.

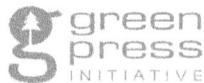